THE

COSMETIC

SURGERY

REVOLUTION

An objective guide to understanding
your cosmetic surgery choices

THE
COSMETIC
SURGERY
REVOLUTION

**An objective guide to understanding
your cosmetic surgery choices**

Robert Scheer with Kathleen O'Connor

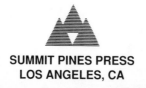

**SUMMIT PINES PRESS
LOS ANGELES, CA**

ISBN: 0-945806-09-4

Cover design by Neasi Design Project.

Printed and bound in the United States of America

SUMMIT PINES PRESS
6399 Wilshire Blvd, #719
Los Angeles, CA 90048

Errata:
Robert Scheer is listed on the back cover as a contributing editio▮
when in fact he is an investigative reporter for the Los Angeles Time▮

To Nina Greene and Stan Burroway, and to Stanley and Betty Sheinbaum and Helen and Pete Zacchino, all of whom have aged beautifully.

—Robert Scheer

CONTENTS

PREFACE

All the publicity about silicone gel breast implants has pointed out a few black holes in the realm of cosmetic plastic surgery.

Most shocking of all is the nearly total lack of legislation. The FDA is just now getting around to testing a product (the implants) that has been on the market for 30 years, although admittedly under the FDA's authority for only a little more than half that time; a product which may result in debilitating diseases or even cancer among many women. And doctors, we discover, are legally allowed to perform brain surgery in their garages if they so choose, since once in the garage they are out of the regulatory jurisdiction of a hospital review staff. Elective, "minor" surgeries such as most cosmetic procedures can easily be performed in outpatient clinics which are as little supervised as private garages. Even insurance companies do not involve themselves with cosmetic surgery regulation, as most cosmetic procedures are not covered in any way by insurance.

Cosmetic plastic surgery simply falls through all of the cracks in terms of safety regulation. It's very much a situation of *caveat emptor:* let the buyer beware. The consumer is not buying a dilapidated house or a lemon of a car, however. The consumer, the cosmetic surgery candidate, is risking his or her looks—and life.

Elective cosmetic plastic surgery for purely aesthetic reasons (pick one of these qualifying terms according to which society your surgeon belongs) is a specialty in a state of flux. The specialty originated in the thirties with official recognition by the American Board of Medical Specialties as Plastic and Reconstructive Surgery. More than ten years ago, another group formed as a regulatory society for doctors who perform strictly cosmetic procedures, the American Board of Cosmetic Surgery, with the theory that the training for certification in plastic and reconstructive surgery is not sufficiently specialized. According to the "plastic," their training gives them a solid knowledge in body and bone structure which a "cosmetic," who may have originally been certified as a dentist or gynecologist, might not possess. To this the "cosmetics" reply that their cosmetic surgeons seek extensive training to perform the procedures for which they are certified. And then the "plastics" want to know whether by "extensive training," do the cosmetics mean a six-hour weekend course?

The fact is, a person with a degree in medicine (any specialty) can buy a liposuction machine in the morning and perform enough procedures by the afternoon to pay for the machine, with pure profit from then on. How well does this MD perform liposuction? Who knows?

The other fact is that many doctors, such as otolaryngologists, do have training in facial surgery. Although they are not eligible to be certified as "plastic" surgeons, they are qualified *and* certified to do facial surgery, and many do it brilliantly (although you might not want to see a nose doctor for your tummy tuck).

The truth is that there are competent surgeons in each group. The cosmetic surgery candidate must be ready to do a lot of research, both into the background of a prospective surgeon and into the facts of the procedure itself. The purpose of this book is to assist the reader in making his or her own informed decisions. We do not propose to recommend or to discourage.

Cosmetic surgery is not for everyone. It is major surgery and should be considered carefully. There are risks of varying gravity. For a person in the right frame of mind, and with the appropriate physiognomy (i.e. a "good" candidate), cosmetic surgery can be the most wonderful gift that person could give to him- or herself.

I have had three personal experiences with plastic/cosmetic surgeons. All occurred in my early twenties when I believed what I was told and when I really didn't have a firm idea of who I was or even who I wanted to be. I was easy prey!

My voice teacher suggested that the inherited circles under my twenty-year-old eyes might keep me from being a success. I didn't even question him about the dubious relationship between the circles under my eyes and my singing voice. I dutifully went to see a surgeon. Twenty minutes and a hundred and fifty dollars later, I was told that the shape of my eyes (big and round) made such surgery extremely difficult to do well. The surgeon told me that I would very likely end up with "round-eye syndrome" in which the lower lid hangs down loosely and exposes the pink inside of the lid. The thought of making my eyes look *worse* instead of better caused me to lose interest. Yet had the surgeon been a little hungrier and not so ethical, who can say what the result would have been?

My aunts used to gloat, "You have the *Williams* behind. It's in our family." They were relieved that they didn't suffer alone. So I saw a surgeon about what I expected to be liposuction, but wasn't; the technique he described was so terrifying that I wanted to flee immediately. It was sort of a series of plugs taken out of your buttocks and thighs, creating a honeycomb effect, then you wear a girdle for three to six months, and the holes heal. To add insult to injury (and I never told my aunts the rest of this), the doctor said that there was too much fat to be removed from my behind, and that I would have to go to the hospital for major surgery called surgical lipectomy. I really didn't want my rear end cut off that badly. What's more, I wear a size 8. Doctors prefer their liposuction candidates to be slim and trim with just a couple of trouble spots such as saddlebags, but how much slimmer than an 8 does one have to be?

Liposuction, described later in this book, uses suction through a tiny pipe called a cannula to remove localized fat deposits from small incisions. You do have to wear a long-legged girdle for several months, and the process does take six months out of your life for full recovery. Liposuction is most effective on skinny women with saddlebags that a thousand years of Rover's Revenge or the Stairmaster won't affect. As fat is suctioned out, so is blood, and to remove too much fat without a blood transfusion is very dangerous.

And what good is it if it won't cure the dreaded Williams Behind in fifteen minutes or less?

My third experience was disturbing. I visited an otolaryngologist about a sore throat. As I was leaving, he said, "Your nose is too wide for your face; have you ever noticed? I can fix it for you. I will put it on your insurance—I'll say you're having trouble breathing." I didn't have insurance, and I hadn't asked for his opinion about my nose. I said I'd think about it, just to be polite. But on the way home I was checking out my nose in the rear-view mirror, saying "Hmmmmm . . . " to myself. I bought right into someone else's assessment of my appearance. Needless to say, if you happen upon a doctor who gives you a pitch like this, run. What he was proposing was not only unethical, it's illegal.

The best doctors will discourage you from surgery if they feel you are not a good candidate. If a doctor advises you against surgery, take heed, even if you decide to go ahead anyway with another doctor. You can be sure that the first doctor is being honest, if only about his or her own capabilities, because he/she is turning down a lucrative procedure.

Choosing a doctor should be the result of a thorough interview process. You should begin with your network of friends and acquaintances, especially those who have had the surgery done with results that you find pleasing. Remember that outpatient surgical facilities are not regulated by any body: neither the government, nor the hospitals, nor the insurance companies—not even by the doctors themselves in a "peer review" system. There is no law. The doctor operating the facility has total control. You will need to have absolute trust in that doctor before you allow him or her to put you to sleep, and to cut you in a way that could be irreparable.

You should interview several doctors. Preliminary consultations cost money, as much as $150 or possibly more. The doctor should spend an hour or more with you in this consultation, as there is much to discuss. Most doctors will apply the fee for the consultation to the fee for the surgery if you go ahead.

Ask about the doctor's hospital affiliations. Get him/her to talk candidly about everything that could go wrong. With any surgery, however minor, there is always the possibility of complications. Beware of a doctor who paints a picture of smooth sailing. If the doctor is not affiliated with an accredited hospital, you may want to reconsider surgery with him. His ability to get you admitted to a hospital *quickly* in the event of complications could mean life or death for you. It's that simple.

Find out what procedure the doctor enjoys the most. This is likely to be the area in which you will see his/her best results. Try to find a surgeon whose favorite procedure is the one you want done. Attend a lecture given by the doctor such as the one I went to given by one of my sources. I noticed that he showed many slides of rhinoplasty and facelifts, and spoke enthusiastically about his techniques and results. When he arrived at the subject of liposuction, however, he had only three or four sets of slides, and spoke very little. Later I asked him directly why he didn't like to do liposuction, and although he was surprised at my observation, he admitted that he found liposuction boring. This man is a brilliant surgeon, an excellent speaker, and a true artist. I would confidently put myself in his hands for facial procedures. But I might look elsewhere for liposuction. After I step-aerobic myself down to a size 2.

Look for a passionate love of the work when you talk to a surgeon. Your surgery is really an artistic endeavor, and your surgeon should think like an artist. You will find that many aesthetic surgeons pursue art in one of its myriad forms as a hobby. Be sure to ask your surgeon to describe how he imagines you will look after the procedure. His/her ideas should agree with yours or you must arrive at a mutual compromise—before anesthesia is administered!

Your surgeon will not be giving you a new face or body, but will be subtly changing your looks for the better. If you bring an unrealistic photo of how you want to look or if you have your heart set on looking like your favorite entertainment personality, STOP. You would be wise to work on accepting yourself as you are, bulges and all, before you opt for surgery. Self-love is blind to physical imperfections.

Have the doctor describe the surgical aspects of the procedure. Doctors will often have photographs of surgery in progress. Before-and-after photographs are interesting and can be helpful if you keep in mind that they are not photographs of *you*—that you are different and that your surgery may turn out differently. If each "after" photo is a carbon copy of the last, however, be warned that the doctor likes one style of this feature (nose or chin, for example), and may not take the composite face or body into consideration. Ask the doctor about his/her worst results. Does he have photos? Is he candid about these cases? No matter how talented a surgeon is, there are always cases which could have come out better.

Ask about recovery: pain, bruising, length of recovery time at home and how long it will take to feel normal again. You may be a quick healer and want to get back to work, or you may feel like taking it easy. Ask the doctor how much help you will need during recovery. If you have no one at home, you might wish to stay at a "hideaway," which is a luxury hospice where you can be cared for in a hotel-like setting. Your doctor may be able to suggest one.

Costs can very widely. *Don't shop for the least expensive*

doctor! Do not base your choice of doctor on the price. You are not buying a car. You are risking your life. You must feel that you can place your life and your looks in your surgeon's hands. You should expect to pay for the surgeon's superior expertise.

Financing is available for elective plastic procedures, which are rarely covered by insurance. Beware of a doctor who says your procedure will be covered by insurance or that he/she will concoct a story. This is known as fraud. The surgeon may have a financing company with whom he/she works.

Most cosmetic procedures turn out very well, and make a lot of people really happy. The decision to change your looks should be carefully considered, however. Why would you risk your life to look better? Why not? How great are the risks, anyway? Well, it is major surgery. You might get more dates. But who wants to get involved with someone who is so superficially interested in looks? Or do you need to get real? It's a jungle out there in the singles scene. For that matter, considering the divorce rate, maybe it's a good idea to keep the marriage rejuvenated along with your face and behind. Isn't true love blind, though?

The only reason to have cosmetic surgery is to please yourself. Although it might take awhile to get used to the changes, you should be more comfortable with the aesthetics of your body after your surgery.

But the *real you* will be the same.

Kathleen O'Connor

ACKNOWLEDGEMENTS

I would like to acknowledge all of the wonderful surgeons, both plastic and cosmetic, who have contributed to this book and who have helped immeasurably to make it a project of which I am very proud. I would particularly like to mention Dr. Lawrence Seifert, whose freedom with his immensely valuable time, his perusal of the finished product, and most importantly, his ability to remain openminded as an advisor even while audibly gritting his teeth as a plastic surgeon, have earned him my eternal gratitude and respect. Others who have graciously taken time out of their extremely busy schedules and who I thank profusely are Dr. John Reinisch of Children's Hospital, Los Angeles, and the University of Southern California; Dr. Julius Newman, President of the American Society of Cosmetic Surgeons; Norma Collier, who represents the California Society of Surgeons; Elizabeth Sadati from the American Society of Aesthetic Plastic Surgeons; Sybil Goldrich of Command Trust Network; nurse-anesthetist Skip Verne; and also Dr. Bruce Achauer of the University of California at San Diego and Dr. David Apfelberg of Palo Alto for the fascinating information on lasers. I would also like to thank all of the contributors in the compilation section who kindly gave us permission to use their work. There is much more excellent information out there which could fill several volumes. We regret not being able to use it all.

I would also like to thank Dodd Darin for his faith, support, and brilliant ideas; Bob Scheer for being Bob Scheer; my parents for raising me right; and all the angels and saints.

Kathleen O'Connor

OVERVIEW

by Robert Scheer

The idea for this book came one afternoon in the operating room of a celebrity surgeon famous for redesigning Joan Rivers' face. I was there to do a series of articles for the Los Angeles Times, and up to that moment the assignment had seemed something of a lark. But suddenly the sight of a woman whose face was being sliced and reordered while the good doctor stanched the considerable flow of blood brought home the harsh reality that while cosmetic surgery is elective it is also quite risky.

Over the next year of research I would discover that while many doctors know what they are doing, others do not; and that the law governing their activities is vague and offers little protection for the consumer considering what are most often major surgical procedures. Nor is it an easy matter for the consumer to pick a competent doctor. Cosmetic surgery is one of the last truly lucrative frontiers of medicine and a fierce turf war between doctors from competing branches of medicine eager to cash in on the prize has muddied the water. Any MD can perform any cosmetic procedure in an outpatient setting virtually free of regulation by either the government or private insurance agencies.

As a result patients have been butchered by incompetent quacks who perform invasive surgery with only the barest of preparation. But while thousands of people have died or been grossly disfigured as the result of bungled procedures we continue to treat this growing field more as a source of humor than as a matter of serious health policy.

The very language of cosmetic or, as some prefer, plastic surgery masks its serious purpose: a major operation cutting into a human to refute the laws of nature. Desirable perhaps, but also potentially dangerous. Yet when friends heard what I was up to, they inevitably lapsed into stand-up comic jokes about face stretches, nose jobs and tummy tucks, as if all that represented some minor joke rather than very serious surgery.

They refused to take the subject seriously, even though in the very next breath I would be asked for the names of the "best" surgeons, since they had "a cousin" or "a friend" who was considering cosmetic surgery. In reality, they were most often getting advice for themselves but were too embarrassed to ask directly. The giddiness of their remarks masked genuine apprehension over what they themselves realized was a deadly serious business. Serious in that all of the cosmetic procedures involve real health risks, including death, and also because life after a major change in one's appearance can produce traumatic results.

The seriousness of cosmetic surgery procedures, although most often glossed over in magazine advertisements, was driven home to me that day in the doctor's operating room. Yes, the man was truly competent, the equipment was of the highest quality, and "The Phantom of the Opera" was playing softly in the background. But on the operating table there was the sight of a naked middle-aged woman with a third of her face flopped over on itself, while the doctor used an electric prod to stem some incidental bleeding. A truly ghastly sight, but apparently no need to worry as he concluded the four-hour ordeal by lifting the skin taut over cheek implants, snipping off patches of excess and cutting a new "V" insert for the ears.

A silicone chin, manufacture size No. 2, was shoved in through the mouth, fat collected from the thigh was shot into the lips for a fuller look and the fifty-something woman now had a forty-something face for only twenty-something thousand dollars.

"What is going on?" I thought. Is nothing about the human makeup inviolate, or are we pieces of material to be cut up and patterned anew? For the surgeons, even the best among them, the answer is that the patients are indeed raw material to be sculpted or patterned into something better than God or Mother Nature intended.

"We treat these conditions, in much the same way you would 'take in' a blouse or dress that is too large, by removing excess material, restitching the garment and ironing out the wrinkles," says the doctor, who can do two or three face lifts a day and who is booked for the next three years.

There you have it. There are cheaper rates, and not every surgeon deals with celebrities, but the public disclosures of facial and body sculpting by the likes of Michael Jackson, Phyllis Diller, Barbara Walters and Cher have set a new standard for the masses and created a multibillion dollar medical industry. This year a million Americans will tamper with the once-immutable laws of physical beauty and aging, availing themselves of cheek, breast and buttock implants, suctioning fat from their thighs and having their noses redesigned and tummies tucked.

What plastic surgeons tend to call "aesthetic" surgery and rival specialists refer to as "cosmetic" surgery has broken through technological, medical and economic barriers to revolutionize expectations for the human body. After a century in which such surgery was a rare art practiced almost clandestinely for the benefit of a few rich clients—mostly high-priced entertainers and socialites—it is now a mass commodity. Like it or not, liberating or grotesque, a cosmetic surgery revolution is upon us and unstoppable.

Even the occasional health scare, such as the recent Food and Drug Administration inquiry into breast implants, seems to have little lasting effect on this lucrative and largely unregulated market.

The prospect of a "New You," as the shingle of one successful Southern California surgeon promises, is now only a matter of a few thousand dollars away. And if cash is a problem, a new nose or breasts can always be charged on the MasterCard.

"There's a waiting list of people who want the surgery that don't have the money." says Dr. Liz Ashley, one of the few women cosmetic surgeons. "They try everything that they can. 'Can I bring you my gold jewelry?' 'Can I give you my pink slip to my car?' 'Can you hold the check three days?' Well, you do the surgery and the check bounces."

Ashley, whose advertising flyer proclaims "Body by Ashley" and promises that "larger fuller breasts can be achieved usually in about one hour," practices in Newport Beach where the competition for the perfect body can be fierce.

"We're so health conscious—and part of it is being able to fill out clothing," says Dr. Malcolm D. Paul, an Orange County California surgeon, contending, in effect, that implant surgery is a logical extension of the fitness craze. Now that the FDA has banned silicone implants the marketing has turned to the sale of saline filled sacs that are presumed to be safer because the body naturally excretes rather than absorbs the saline in the event of a leak. But women still demand the "improvement."

Paul, a member of the American Society of Plastic and Reconstructive Surgeons, says that some prospective candidates for breast enhancement "go to the gym and they see other girls and they get concerned about getting undressed because they are not as full. Of course, the standard is different because some of the girls have had it [breast augmentation] done."

The problem, as Paul indicates, is that the standards keep getting raised. Now women at the health club are attempting to compete with bodies that are often the result of surgery, not exercise.

One result, Paul says, is that, over the years, the "B" cup that was typically requested when he began doing breast enhancements a decade ago has gone to a "C" and increasingly a "D." "In the 1,000 women I have done," he notes, "I've never had one come back and say to me 'They're too large.' "

Demand is somewhat seasonal. A rise in the demand for breast implants coincides with the swimsuit season; face lifts are popular when college reunions near.

"They are dying to go to their reunion to see how everybody looks so old but them," Ashley reports.

The cosmetic surgery boom is being fueled by celebrity endorsements, improved techniques, eroding taboos and declining revenues in other medical specialties. Billions of dollars are involved and in a frenzy of sutures, implants, nips and tucks, the verities of beauty and age are being shattered.

Chemical facial peels and buttock lifts have joined such traditional aids to vanity as cosmetics, fashion and exercise. Once rarely achieved but natural standards of beauty are now routinely replicated in a new tribal tradition in which noses and chins are pulverized to make way for the reconstruction of that which is smaller, straighter, upturned or indented. No one need be plain; patients often appear with clipped photos of stunning magazine models, expecting the same for themselves.

Anything is possible—almost.

"To the limits of surgical ability, you can really change a lot," Paul observed, "But you have to have a good underlying bony structure, especially in the face. In the breasts it's amazing how you can change around not only small breasts to larger, but asymmetrical breasts. . . . It's a very rapidly changing field. The other day I did a body contour, breast, plus nose, all on the same gal. It took about four hours to do everything. She went home well motivated."

The transformation of physical appearance—formerly relegated to National Geographic Magazine layouts about stretching lips and the like in what were thought of as more primitive cultures—is now the subject of high medical science and physicians' whims.

"Patients say this is what God gave me, now I want you to do better," says a leading Newport Beach facial plastic surgeon, adding, "You are working in the most precious medium of all art. You are doing living art on living human tissue."

Perhaps, but sometimes in the process the aesthetically exotic has been rendered commercial and mechanical.

In his Irvine, California, office, dermatologist and surgeon Dr. Jeffrey Alan Klein, a widely published expert, draws crude circles dissected by lines on the inner thighs and buttocks of women in preparation for liposuction. Looking very much like the graffiti symbols of underground cults, the lines in the circle are intended to guide the metal rod probing under the skin sucking up blood and fat to be passed through tubes to collection jars.

Klein, who has pioneered one of the more widely used techniques of liposuction, is proud that he works with patients who are under local anesthesia. He reasons that an alert patient will warn a doctor who probes too deeply, perhaps threatening to puncture the kidney or some other vital organ, as has happened in other surgeons' offices.

Offices like Klein's are popping up everywhere, particularly in California, New York and Florida, and are now threatening to be as common to mini-mall life as fast food outlets. Plastic surgery is elective, and is generally not covered by insurance, so it is free from most supervision and can be performed in out-patient facilities. And anyone with an M.D. degree can do it no matter their specialty training or lack thereof.

The enormous profitability of elective cosmetic surgery has resulted in a frenetic turf war between plastic surgeons, who are certified by the American Board of Plastic Surgery, and an increasing number of other specialists—gynecologists, dermatologists, ophthalmologists—who contend that they are equally qualified to perform such procedures.

A few blocks from dermatologist Klein one finds the "New You Plastic Surgery" office of plastic surgeon Martin P. Elliott, who tends to stress the distance between his world and that of the other specialists who have entered the field. Whereas Klein uses before-and-after pictures to advertise in slick magazines, Elliott restricts himself to a conservative print ad in the yellow pages. But Elliott and Klein are clearly in the same business, and fishing in the same pool for customers.

Whatever the differences in doctors' training, it remains very much a commercial business, as one is reminded in Elliott's "New You" consulting room where a score of new breast implants, squiggly and quite sensuous in their own right, are spread out over a layer of past issues of *Playboy* and *Cosmopolitan*, along with the standard industry brochures describing nipple placement, fat vacuuming, buttock lifting, pectoral implants, face lifts, nose reconstruction and the other achievements of the modern art of live body sculpture.

Elliott, a respected plastic surgeon, seems a bit embarrassed by the "New You" sign over his office but has resigned himself to salesmanship. What the consumer/patient needs to remember is that this is after all a business. We are talking here about healthy patients volunteering to make themselves temporarily ill and risk injury or death for appearance's sake. The doctors who succeed at it are the ones who are the better salesmen. The hype of the customer, which rubs up against one of the basic canons of medicine—do no harm—is inevitable. The alternative, simply performing fine medical work, doesn't bring in the customers. As Elliott recalls:

"When I started out, I covered 12 emergency rooms. I worked every night. I stitched people up and they came back to the office and I did a lot of hand surgery and I did this and I did that. I became known as the best reconstructive surgeon in the area. It didn't bring one single cosmetic surgery patient into my office.

"All the guys down at the beach were busy cultivating the cosmetic surgery patients and talking to some ladies' society. I wasn't doing any of that. It was time to change, and I got wise, too. The bottom line is that unless you do some form of self-aggrandizement, you don't get the work. It's like the phone book ad, the TV commercial. Businesses that want to be successful, advertise."

The market incentive is pervasive, as respected surgeons vie in advertising before-and-after pictures of the bodies they have worked over, often implying that the major surgery involved is painless and risk-free. Competition is so fierce, media exposure so crucial, that many doctors are represented by professional public relations agencies.

"There's dollars and cents involved here," says Thomas R. Stephenson, a West Los Angeles surgeon whose breast implant ads featuring bosomy women in negligees run frequently in The Times, "and you're going to have fellows figuring out ways to get the public to come to them rather than go any place else."

But can one trust the advice of doctors driven by such blatant material incentives? If most of them move into the cosmetic field to make money rather than out of a desire to heal patients can one really expect the physicians to offer objective advice? For example, to counsel that someone might be better off staying just as they are?

After all, a large nose or small breast does not emit a measurable indication of infection or other illness, like taking the temperature or counting the white cells of an ill patient. The incentive here, given the enormous monies involved, is to counsel surgery when it is not needed. We are not talking here about obvious deformities which most in the medical profession and outside would recommend improving. By definition cosmetic surgery means improving a normal appearance. What's to stop a greedy surgeon from recommending surgery to those with even the most imperceptible distance from Hollywood standards of beauty? Very often in visits to doctors' offices I would be introduced to patients who seemed to me to be in every way smashing in their looks before surgery. Yet they were advised to let the surgeon tinker with their appearance and at very high prices.

In fact, even by medical profession standards, the payoff can be enormous. Surgeons in Southern California can easily earn over $1 million a year; it's obvious that doing even a face lift a day for a $15,000 fee can send that figure much higher. What is more, this is money "up front"—offered from the private stash of patients who do not have to await the approval of insurance providers.

If the surgeons and their public relations agents can be believed, most patients will be pleased with the results, cheerfully hock themselves to the hilt, be generally oblivious to the real risks in what is, after all, major surgery, and emerge grateful that their features now conform to a surgeon's notion of beauty. For many patients it is a big but compelling decision—an obsession to look better can suddenly be fulfilled.

"I'm still being asked if I'm glad I did it," Vida Dean, 65, fashion and beauty writer for the Newport Beach/Costa Mesa Pilot, wrote of her face lift last year. "Who would not be glad to have the bags gone from over and under the eyes; have the saggy jowls gone? Any regrets? Oh, yes. Why didn't I do it 10 years ago?"

I must say, that after lunching with this woman, she seemed an otherwise sensible and interesting women who had somehow, perhaps because she covered the society beat, come to be obsessed with maintaining a youthful appearance. But it just was no longer possible to do that, surgery or no, and instead of comfortably settling into old age she fell for the siren song of the surgeons.

But I understand the appeal. Who wouldn't want to shave twenty years off their age or look just like some media star? The fact that it can't really be done will not stop most people from trying and indeed deluding themselves that the desired results have been attained. But at the core of this desperation is a deep-rooted contempt for one's self.

Given the proliferation and power of American media

throughout the world, the implications are enormous for imposing a worldwide standard of beauty. Thanks to cosmetic surgery, people everywhere, if they can afford it, can now order up the eyes, cheekbones or breasts of their favorite North American television star.

Turning a Japanese housewife, for example, into a typical product of the dominant white American genetic mix, is—for whatever that is worth—now eminently doable.

"When I was in Japan, I wanted to be like an American," said a patient of the Newport Beach surgeon. "You know. Big eyes. Everybody, all my girlfriends did their eyes deeper, so I did. ". . . What was she having done now? "Nose and chin this time around." Eyelids are often redone. Asian women don't have a crease in the middle. Why does one need an extra fold like two tracks running horizontally across the eyelid? Why is the smooth expanse of eyelid skin not perfect enough? The answer is that the desirable eye, the one extolled in the massive cosmetic industry blitz campaigns, is the Western eye, and the two lines provide the border for eye shadow and other makeup applications.

What is to be made of all this? Apart from the issue of breast implant safety there has been surprisingly little discussion about what might be regarded as the transmogrification of the human appearance. Since most of the customers—at least 85%—are women, is this not yet another assault on a woman's independence?

Not according to *Ms.* magazine when it celebrated Cher, one of the main role models of the surgeon's designer-body movement. Cher, who has appeared in ads for Jack La Lanne health spas, admits her body comes from "La Lanne and La Knife" and her plastic surgery has been the subject of photo essays and feature stories in magazines and television throughout the world. Yet she is celebrated in the July 1988 issue of *Ms.* precisely for having taken hold of her life in part by employing surgeons who took hold of her body.

"Her message is loved and needed: You can change a lot in

your lifetime, and be . . . honest, and who you really are," says Gloria Steinem.

"With a little help from plastic surgeons, Cher has done wonders with exercise. But we love her just the same," Flo Kennedy, the feminist, is quoted in the same issue.

Oddly enough, this blasé view of plastic surgery ignored a devastating article in *Ms.* just the month before by Sybil Goldrich, a doctor's wife who documented her disastrous experiences with breast implants.

Though the majority of operations may cause no complications, serious problems and even horror stories about cosmetic surgery abound—from breasts that painfully encapsulate to face lifts that produce muscle paralysis.

But, whatever the actual risks, the lines for these procedures are ever longer and the word of mouth from most patients seems to be exultation at bursting onto the scene bustier, younger and, in some cases, more Anglo-American.

The concern about various aspects of plastic surgery expressed by those who claim to be victims and by public interest groups has been overwhelmed by the gushing enthusiasm of show business celebrities.

"I'm a walking billboard for cosmetic surgery," said Phyllis Diller last year. "At 73, I look a red-hot 50, so I think it's great."

With the stars setting the standard, it's no wonder that their fans have followed uncritically. Patients interviewed often mention the lips of actress Barbara Hershey in the movie "Beaches," or television personality Barbara Walters' candid discussion of her face lift.

"You start watching television and you start looking at these people. Like these news commentators," said Barbara Pigeon. "You think, 'What have these people done?'" Pigeon, who worked in a surgeon's office, was inspired by the example of the TV newscasters to have her eyes done, and much more.

"I had a breast operation first, about five years ago. I was older, I had never had children, I was not very well-endowed . . . I just wanted to be a little bit bigger. I did not want to be the broad on the beach. I wanted to be more aesthetic looking. None of the clothes fit properly." She now is rather busy and says she has never had any medical problems as a result of her surgery.

Her husband followed suit, "He had his waist 'lipo'ed'. I had to take all his pants in to the cleaners to be altered."

The motivation for cosmetic surgery most often cited by women is that they want clothes to fit right, and indeed the demand for cosmetic surgery is highest in those areas that also are given to a greater preoccupation with fashion, such as Southern California, New York and Florida.

Stephenson, the West Los Angeles surgeon, mentions that he has a doctor friend in Anchorage to whom he taught his technique of breast enhancement, making the friend a top expert in Anchorage. But, by Southern California standards, the Anchorage surgeon's business is very slow. "He's done five a month. I could do two a day," said Stephenson, who charges $5,000 for the procedure, and says he has performed 3,000 implant operations.

Stephenson explains the interest in fashion and the body that is needed to go with it: "Face it, women are dolled up for us."

This matter-of-fact condescension is typical of the male surgeons, many of whom tend to refer to women patients, including some aged sixty, as "girls."

Surgeons also engage in a form of "outing," discreetly dropping names to a reporter of prominent persons they claim have benefited from procedures they offer. They scoff at the notion that aging is to be accepted or that its visible proof, like lines in the face, might be an indication of maturity, wisdom or attractiveness. Most of the surgeons interviewed were themselves less than perfect in appearance and showed some signs of aging, but none had availed themselves of the opportunities for a cut-rate face lift.

"The only way to age gracefully is with cosmetic surgery," says the prominent Newport Beach surgeon, who could be described as youthful-looking. He says he is willing to undergo such surgery himself at some point and observes that his face lift clientele now is 15% male.

In a recent operation in the doctor's office a man who seemed to be over sixty was indeed having the fat sacs scraped from under the skin around his eyes. But, even if such extensive surgery went well, it was clear from viewing his body on the operating table that the aging process would not easily be reversed.

One problem at the outset is how much to alter. For example, another patient in the office, a woman also in her sixties, had recently had her face lifted, fat removed from her eyelids, a chin implant and a "nose correction" but clearly still looked less than young. She volunteered that for the time being she would resist having chemical peels to remove her wrinkles. "I don't want to become a plastic surgery junkie," she said.

In any case, cosmetic surgery is not a stable solution to the aging process. Most surgeons, while they are proud of their results, concede that they are not permanent, and that periodic and costly tuneups are called for, lest gravity and other natural effects have their way. For example, collagen injections to the face to give it a more youthful look last less than four months.

Sometimes this has led to the use of questionable procedures. Some surgeons have been injecting silicone directly into the face as an alternative to the temporary effects of collagen. Silicone is indeed permanent, so much so that if it is misapplied or shifts it can result in disfigurement.

Because silicone is a product, the federal Food and Drug Administration has regulatory authority over its use, and last year it intervened to ban the sale of silicone for facial injections. But there is no comparable regulation by any government authority over the techniques, skills and training required of physicians performing cosmetic surgery procedures.

Instead, there are competing advertising campaigns conducted by the more aggressive surgeons, which many professionals in the field believe confused and trivialized the serious choices confronting patients. Physicians have been allowed to advertise, since a 1979 decision of the Federal Trade Commission, which treated medical advertisements as no different than those for other consumer services.

Extensive advertising in the trendier magazines, together with the celebrity endorsements, has created an aura that renders cosmetic surgery both respectable and inevitable, and many in the field expect it to be as common as orthodontics in the near future. In some circles, it is even now an expected aspect of the successful lifestyle. Often, surgery so selective tends to be packaged as something that is both healthful and a requirement for success.

That was the theme, for example, of a 1981 article in the magazine *The Executive* by Dr. Robert Kotler, who extolled face lifts as a way for male executives to meet the oncoming competition of "well-educated minorities and newly liberated, ambitious women" by eliminating "any signs of fatigue or slowdown."

Kotler, who is a faculty member at UCLA and a consultant to the Medical Board of California, did not mention any medical risk in connection with the face lift procedures and peels he advocated. Nor was there a hint that this might not be for everyone.

"While other societies and cultures may venerate the aged, ours prefers to emphasize agelessness," Kotler wrote, in an article he now says has become "a classic."

The article included a catalogue of possible surgeries, along with advice to corporations to include cosmetic surgery in their executive incentive programs as a way of improving productivity. Implying that those offered surgery really ought to go along, Kotler wrote, "Even if the executive does not see the value of improved appearance, his company might." Why? Simply because, "Regardless of how well they are functioning they also have to look like they are functioning well."

Some surgeons insist on a less aggressive marketing approach. They stress that the procedures are not for everyone and warn their patients not to expect too much change in their lives, personal or professional, as a result of the surgery.

Lawrence N. Seifert, a Los Angeles surgeon and spokesman for the American Society for Aesthetic Plastic Surgery, for example, has turned away patients "because they weren't ready." He spends considerable time with patients discussing the pros and cons of the procedure, sometimes more than in the actual operation. He is not alone in stressing that this is major surgery that ought to be carefully considered.

The need for such caution seems obvious when one realizes that the vast majority of such operations are performed in a doctor's office outside of the purview of state and federal regulatory agencies.

Under such circumstances, "No minimum standards exist either for doctors, for their staff to assist them or for the facilities in which they operate," Frank A. Papineau, a congressional investigator, concluded after a four year study. Papineau, of the House Committee on Small Business, added that "No certification process exists to give consumers a true idea of whether the physician is actually qualified to perform a given procedure, no requirements exist even for the basic life-support equipment in these office-based surgeries. Doctors in their medical facilities are not required to have medical malpractice insurance, and we found far too many did not." Most surgeons agree on the need for increased regulation, but they remain jealous of their medical prerogatives and divided over which way to proceed.

While cosmetic or aesthetic surgery may be an enormous boon to some patients, it has been a disaster for others, and many health care professionals fear that there is little reason to expect the two types of patients and the two types of doctors— competent and not—to be carefully sorted out in today's over-heated market.

The problem is that the field is largely unregulated and today's much sought-after surgeon might prove to be tomorrow's reject. That was the case with Dr. Elam, one of the most famous and successful of Southern California's cosmetic surgeons.

I well remember the adulation visited upon this doctor during his prime. The scene was set in Newport Beach at a very tony charity bash back in 1986 and the suave, good-looking doctor was the star of the night. After all, he had created Phyllis Diller's much publicized new face and the star had been positively gushing in her praise of the doctor who had made her look, she claimed, "twenty years younger." Many of Newport's wealthiest had followed her path to the fountain of youth at Elam's office and most were quite pleased with the results.

That night at the auction they clapped as Elam stood and pointed out some of the proud beneficiaries of his work in the audience and several women rose, taut of face with augmented chests held high, to reveal medical miracles that are now routinely performed, and, to the approving crowd that night, apparently risk-free.

But five years later Elam's license to practice medicine was revoked, in a rare action by the Medical Board of California, on charges of malpractice and insurance fraud.

The case reveals a growing split in the medical community over safety, standards and ethics in the largely unregulated field of cosmetic surgery. Elam, a past president of the American Society of Cosmetic Surgery (the "cosmetics"), claims he was done in by a rival medical faction—members of the American Society of Plastic and Reconstructive Surgery (the "plastics")—in an unseemly battle over what may be modern medicine's largest pot of gold.

"I'm the victim of a turf war over who has the right to perform cosmetic surgery, which is the most lucrative field in medicine," says Elam, who is appealing the case. "It's the last place that we have independence because, since it's elective surgery, we're not under the dictum of a hospital, insurance company, or other outside groups."

To some, that's just the problem. Cosmetic surgery, largely elective and performed in outpatient settings, is strikingly free of regulation either by the government or by the private sector. As a result, virtually any such surgery may be performed by the holder of an MD license no matter what his or her specialization, making it difficult to establish common standards. As the Elam case illustrates, consumers of the doctor's services are buffeted by competing and bewildering claims of competency. Judging who is right for the job is no easy matter when highly trained doctors deny their competitors' credentials, basing their critiques largely on the fact that the other fellow is not a member of their chosen medical society.

The expert witnesses against Elam were "plastics" who had completed a residency and passed boards in general plastic surgery. They claimed Elam botched a tummy tuck, gave a patient cheek implants she did not want, and fraudulently described operations as medically necessary in order to claim insurance payments. "He changed a Mrs. America runner-up into a recluse who hides in her house," claims Dr. Robert Minor, a "plastic" who was the chief medical witness for the state.

Scores of physicians, most of them "cosmetics," meaning that their surgical training was in branches of medicine other than plastic surgery, have rallied to Elam's defense. They contend that the case against him was based on two old complaints out of 5,000 operations over ten years, that the insurance company did not challenge his claims, and that the dissatisfied patient went on to win the Mrs. California contest— after her surgery. Elam, who is board-certified as an ear, nose and throat specialist, argues bitterly that patients have died following plastic surgery performed by "plastics" without any official consequences.

The internecine warfare among medical specialties has led to a bewildering array of claims to legitimacy that must be sorted out, without government guidance, by potential patients who often have limited knowledge of the serious risks involved.

"Untold numbers of patients seeking the fountain of youth

through a face lift, a tummy tuck or an acid peel sometimes get more than they bargained for," Rep. Ron Wyden (D-Ore.) warned last April at a hearing of the subcommittee on regulation of the House Committee on Small Business. "Suffering, infection, stroke and occasionally death [follow] procedures that are advertised as safe, easy and painless."

As Wyden's statement suggests, the medical questions associated with cosmetic surgery go far beyond the much-publicized issues of the safety of breast implants, which the Food and Drug Administration has recently been investigating. The FDA has jurisdiction only over medical products, not over physicians' medical practices. Neither the FDA nor any other government agency, state or federal, regulates the surgical work of physicians or the clinical setting in which it is done.

For most surgery, such regulation is provided largely by the standards set by hospital boards and by the insurance companies that pay for it. But 80% of cosmetic surgery is performed in doctors' own clinics and other outpatient settings where hospital regulation does not apply. And since most cosmetic surgery is not insured, doctors have no need to prove to insurance companies that patients are ill and in need of medical treatment. In fact, cosmetic surgery involves the reverse—making healthy people temporarily unwell—and it is being performed today by doctors who may or may not be trained adequately for the procedures involved, often in office operating rooms that are not required to meet even the sanitary codes demanded of a doughnut shop.

"[In] restaurants, the facility, the kitchen, the whole thing, probably even the width of the door, is subject to all kinds of regulations," observes Kenneth J. Wagstaff, executive director of the Medical Board of California. "But there's no productive way that the government has of telling the doctor this is how to have a sterile office, how he shall train his staff."

In California, in fact, the definition of a doctor's office is vague enough to include square-block facilities that look like small hospitals. As long as the MD claims it as his or her office, the state accepts that definition, even if it contains multiple operating rooms.

As a result, Wagstaff says, "there currently is no legal requirement for either licensure, peer review or accreditation" for outpatient surgery in California. He adds that plastic, cosmetic and liposuction procedures "are routinely performed in small clinics or private physicians' offices . . . In these situations, there may be no quality assurance other than the physician's own self-regulation."

Nationally, this loophole in regulation has been documented in detail during three years of hearings by Wyden's House subcommittee, but during all that time the committee has not managed to introduce a bill to curtail abuses. The opposition by the powerful medical lobby, with influential physician members in every congressional district, has been fierce, according to a committee staff member.

Wyden observes that the vast majority of physicians "are honest, decent and caring. But for the significant minority who aren't, outpatient or free-standing clinics are a natural place to set up shop. The lack of peer review, accreditation procedures, training requirements, or even minimal quality assurance programs give questionable medical providers an open field to ply their trade."

Wyden cited one case in which a Southern California doctor allowed his bookkeeper to administer general anesthesia during an office surgery. The patient died. The doctor broke no law, because his MD license makes him the law in his own office. In a second instance, a doctor whose training in chemical face peels consisted of only a week-long seminar, "cooked" the patient's skin and left her appearing "like a monster." Another witness before the committee had suffered a stroke after an unqualified surgeon performed a tummy-tuck.

But who is "qualified?" Current law provides no guidelines other than the requirement of an MD license.

"It is perfectly legal in this country for a dermatologist to do brain surgery in his garage if he can find a patient that is willing

to get on the table and pay for it," says Frank A. Papineau.
Wagstaff, of the state medical board agrees: "If you are an MD,
under law technically read, you can do anything."

Brain surgery, however, probably would not be performed
in a garage or even an office operating room because the
insurance companies or Medicare would not pay for it. Standards
for most non-elective outpatient surgery are set indirectly by
the agencies that must meet the bills. That would extend to all
the requirements for a safe surgical environment. But most
cosmetic surgery, being uninsured, is free of such restraints.

Historically, the medical profession has justified the wide
latitude doctors are given as a natural perquisite of their
training. The doctor is presumed to be the knowledgeable and
ultimate authority concerning what transpires in his or her
operating room. But with the recent proliferation of out-patient
surgery, an increasing number of physicians have called for
government regulation.

Some surgeons voluntarily apply for accreditation for their
offices from private organizations that offer a measure of
supervision. But many do not and none are required to.
According to Dr. Gustavo Colon, the president of the American
Association for Accreditation of Ambulatory Plastic Surgery
Facilities, an umbrella group attempting to provide such accreditation:

"Even tattoo artists, hairdressers and manicurists need licensing and/or health board examination to practice their
specific art, while a physician who decides to perform surgery
in his office currently does not need licensing for any specific
procedure."

[Editor's note: This regulatory group was established by,
and is available only to plastic surgeons certified by the ASPRS-
KO]

Doctors who defend self-regulation respond that they are
themselves held responsible, being liable to lawsuits, loss of
license and even criminal penalties if something goes awry.
They cite their extensive training, residencies, and peer group

certification by academic, state and professional boards, as justification of their authority.

The problem, critics argue, is that in the area of cosmetic surgery, there is no standard test of knowledge and accomplishment to which all must adhere.

In this rapidly evolving field, some procedures have been popularized after many physicians completed their medical training. A weekend course in the midst of a ski excursion sometimes suffices for formal training in what are complex and potentially dangerous procedures.

While it is legally permissible, should a gynecologist augment breasts, a dermatologist lift the face or an ear nose and throat specialist be engaged in liposuction? Who are entitled to call themselves cosmetic or plastic surgeons?

Surgeons certified by the American Board of Plastic Surgery are adamant in insisting that they are the only ones entitled by virtue of their specialized training to the designation "plastic surgeon." Indignant about the sudden rush of physicians from other specialties into what they feel is their domain, these surgeons, who belong to the American Society of Plastic and Reconstructive Surgeons, have fought a well-financed campaign to expose what they consider to be the sham credentialing of their rivals.

Other specialists: dermatologists, ophthalmologists and otolaryngologists (ear, nose and throat doctors), for example— tend to be grouped in societies bearing the designation "cosmetic" rather than "plastic" or "aesthetic." They strike back with the claim that they are often certified by their own recognized specialty boards, and that they have indeed received advanced training in this field and may have more operating room experience.

For example, ear, nose and throat surgeons argue that they are more qualified to do a nose "correction" than plastic surgeons whose training is more general.

These issues are not easily resolved. Liposuction, an amazingly popular procedure in which fat is sucked out of offensive bulges, is now often being performed by physicians with limited training, and there have been cases in which injuries to vital organs occurred or too much fat was removed. But when plastic surgeons contend that they alone should perform the procedure, others point out that liposuction was pioneered in the '70s by a French abortionist and popularized in this country by "cosmetic" surgeons.

Dermatologists claim liposuction as their natural area of expertise, relating as it does to the fatty tissue under the skin, rather than to underlying structure. Plastic surgeons, though most were not trained in the discipline as students, scoff at that and profess themselves frightened at the idea of people of limited surgical training cutting into the body.

The plastic surgeons have found allies for their claims that problems arise from specialists in other fields exaggerating their competence. For example, Wagstaff of the state medical board says that in one instance a Los Angeles physician who advertised himself as a "board certified" specialist in "plastic reconstruction" was, in fact, an ear, nose and throat doctor with "little advanced training in plastic surgery." The result, Wagstaff says, was that "he disfigured several people and killed one."

Wagstaff adds that he finds the designation "board certified" meaningless because "An American Society of 'Cosmetic This-or-That' or International College of 'Whatchamacallit' that has no rigorous training requirements may form a nonprofit corporation and 'certify' whom they please." But some leading cosmetic surgeons reply that they consider Wagstaff and the state board to be overly influenced by the plastic surgeons' well-financed lobby.

The case for the "plastics" is made by Dr. Martin P. Elliott, a plastic surgeon in Orange County who served seven years of internships and residency in his field and who is certified by the American Board of Plastic Surgery.

"Yes, of course there's a tremendous amount of inferior work. There's a tremendous amount of work being done under less than ideal conditions," he says. "We have dermatologists and general practitioners and chiropractors; everybody's trying to do plastic surgery. There's no way to absolutely prevent it because this is a field where you can do the surgery outside of the hospital environment for the most part and there is no regulation whatsoever."

The counter-argument is that plastic surgeons like Elliott are simply attempting to corner a lucrative market.

That is the view of a past president of the American Academy of Cosmetic Surgery, who wishes to remain anonymous. This organization allegedly is competing with the plastic surgeons' group in which Elliott is active.

This highly successful cosmetic surgeon points out that as an ear, nose and throat specialist, he is certified by a board accredited by the American Medical Association before the plastic surgery board even existed. He argues that cosmetic surgery of the face, particularly rhinoplasty (nose construction) is definitely covered in his training and falls logically within his expertise.

"For a while everybody minded their own business and behaved in a professional, ethical manner and did the plastic surgery that relates to their domain. But the plastic surgeons started a war and they had a very well-thought-out plan," he says. "There are great dermatologists and there are great plastic surgeons and there are lousy plastic surgeons. It is not as clear an issue as everybody would like it to be. These people always look at the opposition as if they were fighting a war"

He backs up his charge with a reference to a "White Paper" issued in 1988 by the then-executive director of the American Society of Plastic and Reconstructive Surgeons. The language of the memorandum has the ring of guerrilla warfare:

"We must plan a course of action that will allow us to stall as long as we can, neutralize their leadership . . . In short, our plan must consist of a stalling mechanism that will force all of their efforts into one level. On another level we must make it appear that we are working with them to improve their educational and knowledge background . . . This appearance must be presented to members of the out group . . . ."

The plastic surgeons' association now claims the paper was the product of one man, who has since been dismissed.

The anonymous Newport Beach cosmetic surgeon charges that the plastic surgeons are attempting to create an unwarranted monopoly, using a propaganda campaign and pressure on state legislators.

"There are so many well-trained, board-certified plastic surgeons who have lost patients," he says. "For example, a doctor in Oakland did a liposuction and she happened to pierce the liver and the spleen and the lung and so on. There is a plastic surgeon in Beverly Hills who put a muscular implant inside the chest! I could go on and on . . . . They have this notion that they are ordained by some super power to be able to do all the surgery that they think is needed and that they have no human frailty. That's bull."

However, the California legislature in its only action to date to regulate this field, adopted standards for advertising proposed by the "plastic" surgeons, which the other organization of "cosmetics" opposed as an arbitrary restraint of trade. Beginning in January of 1993, only board-certified plastic surgeons will be able to advertise themselves as such. [Editor's note: the languaging of this legislation is being debated. The possibility of "equivalent" certification is being allowed and as of this writing, criteria for equivalency is being decided upon. The term "board-certified" therefore may include cosmetic surgeons in the not-too-distant future. Please refer to Senate Bill 2036 in the appendix—KO].

Whatever its merits, the new California law is the first step toward re-regulation of medical advertising. Nationally, such regulation has been largely suspended during the past decade and that has led to a barrage of aggressive ads that now inundate local magazines and reach into mainstream newspapers.

They generally feature photos of women's breasts and buttocks in before and after poses, and often imply that the procedures involved are painless and risk-free. Every surgeon interviewed agreed that was misleading as a description of major surgery, but often their own advertising belied their concern for accuracy.

Not surprisingly, cosmetic surgeons, who are certified by their own medical boards, have been critical of the new law. "There is an intense political effort on the part of the plastic surgeons to inhibit dermatologists from getting any kind of surgical privileges," says Dr. Jeffrey Klein of Irvine, a dermatologist who pioneered a widely used liposuction procedure. "Their argument is that dermatologists don't have surgical training. Forty per cent of dermatology is, in fact, surgical."

Klein, who uses local anesthesia in liposuctions and even in face lifts, defends his procedures as safer than the full anesthesia employed by the plastic surgeons. He argues that anesthesia is the cause of most problems in surgery and that the risks have been "hushed up."

"The complications in outpatient facilities, which is where most cosmetic procedures take place, are a result of anesthesia leading to cardiac problems. How many of these guys [the plastic surgeons] know how to read an EKG, let alone take care of a cardiac arrest?"

Klein has been attempting to track deaths from plastic surgery procedures but finds it difficult to obtain the necessary data because "deaths in ambulatory surgery settings are not reportable in California, so we don't know what the causes are. The coroner gets it, but it's not reportable to the state. The only way to dig out all that data is to go to every coroner's office and to ask them for the records of all the deaths that have occurred."

"I know one doctor in Orange County who had a patient who died two days after a face lift. It was hushed up. That happens all the time throughout California, throughout the nation, but it's not reportable, but whatever the cause of that was, we just don't know."

In a letter sent to Klein, in April of 1990, the Board's chief of enforcement wrote: "I regret that the Medical Board of California does not compile statistical data concerning deaths which occur during ambulatory surgery . . . I am at a loss to suggest another source where you might find the data you seek."

As Klein's remarks indicate, the civil war between the plastic surgeons and their competitors has produced a climate marked by wild charges of incompetency, claims of omniscience and enormous confusion for the patient.

"What has happened now is that the public really cannot rely on board certification anymore," says Elliott. "In order to create a board, all you have to do is incorporate yourself and call it a board."

There does seem to be general agreement that self-regulation has failed and that there is a need for government standards for both physicians and their operating rooms. "It's my feeling that within the next five years we will have regulation," says Elliott. "I'm welcoming it with open arms. This is a situation where people say, 'Well, you haven't regulated yourselves.' We are unable to regulate ourselves, we have been legislated out of the ability to regulate ourselves. Every time we try we get shot down. The argument is that it's a turf war for money. I suppose that is a portion of it, but there is the other aspect of it—that you shouldn't be doing something for which you don't have the training."

The confusion about what is valid training makes it extremely difficult for the patients in this exploding market to decide intelligently about which procedures and practitioners are safe and wise. Clearly, just calling for accuracy in advertising, as the California legislature did, does little to solve the overall problem of regulating an aggressive medical industry that appears to be driven by a gold rush fever.

Of course we now know that this push for the buck became overwhelming in the area of breast implants. Over a period of twenty years millions of women throughout the world had their breasts altered. Yet it took twenty years of breast implant history before the FDA finally moved.

It is important to recognize that the FDA was able to move

against the manufacturers of implants only because it has jurisdiction over medical products. Neither the FDA nor any other federal agency has effective power over the licensing and practice of doctors. For example, attempts to establish national standards for accrediting doctors and regulating their outpatient facilities have never made it out of congressional committee, let alone into law. The medical lobby is just too powerful for that. In the case of implants the government did act, but not against the doctors, who are still free to put anything they can get their hands on into a woman's body.

The breast implant controversy is not over. The FDA has in effect delivered a temporary restraining order until the drug companies prove their products safe. Some have gone out of business rather than face a swarm of lawsuits. Others continue to produce non-silicone implants which remain legal.

Ironically, the breast operation was one of the safer cosmetic surgery procedures and the overwhelming majority of women were, by most accounts, satisfied with their new breasts. And why shouldn't they be? Our society has made such an obsessive fetish of large breasts that a woman with less is bound to feel great pressure to do something to fill out clothes whether it's stuffing stockings in a bra or implants under her skin. As with all cosmetic procedures one ought to be sympathetic with the patient, male or female, who feels the need to conform to society's standard. I have much hair but I can see why so many millions of men go in for transplants. And, because of our double standard which requires the women to be physically attractive while a man need only be interesting, for a woman the size of her breasts has to be a bigger concern than hair for a man. This point was driven home for me in a conversation with a thirty-year-old law student who had a breast job some seven years ago.

"Hoping to meet guys," Sue and her friend Gail were driving to Palm Springs for a mini-vacation. "We were laughing about men and what they liked," Sue recalls, "and in the process I made a couple of flat jokes about my breasts or the lack thereof."

Suddenly the conversation turned serious and Gail said, "You can fix that if you want to, you know—I did." Sue surveyed Gail's breasts and was impressed: "They were wonderful—and just what I wanted! I took the name of her doctor and, two weeks later, I had new breasts, too."

That simple.

Now, eight years later, Sue's breasts have hardened somewhat despite the exercises she performed in the privacy of the company rest room, an inconvenience cheerfully accepted: "Your breasts don't feel as 'normal,' but they look great."

Yes, she is alarmed by sensational news reports of silicone leaking into the body from the implants. Nor can she understand why the Food and Drug Administration only now, two million altered women later, is requiring the manufacturers to prove their products safe.

She also knows that an implant can interfere with the detection of breast cancer through mammography, but has been told that some radiologists have developed compensating techniques.

She admits that she experienced more post-operative pain and inconvenience than she had been led to expect.

And she is angry that her doctor attempted to collect on a fraudulent insurance claim in her case and was not forthcoming about the risks and pain involved.

Having said all that, Sue regrets only not having gone for a larger size.

"If, after I have kids, I have to go through this experience again to even them out," she says, "people are going to notice. This time, I'll take the C's please."

Sue, an aerospace project manager who didn't want her real name used for fear of embarrassment at work, is not silly or frivolous—but neither are breasts in this culture. She is merely being candid about the enduring torment of women forced to measure up to the dominant fashion fetish of their time. "You worry a bit about what's inside of you that's not natural, but you trade that off for looking good in a bikini and having cleavage," she said.

A common choice these days. In fact, future archaeologists digging up millions of non-biodegradable silicone sacs along with silicone chins, cheeks, buttocks and dozens of other implants might well mark it as a distinguishing feature of the era.

After all, women's breasts used to be or not be. They could be pushed up, padded, or in other ways exaggerated to satisfy the demands of fashion and male obsession, but the breast itself was thought to be immutable. Then along came a multibillion dollar medical industry promoting the creation of precisely that size and shape the client might desire—for a price.

"When you get your breasts done and you pay, $3,000, $4000, it's not that much," observes Irvine plastic surgeon Dr. Malcolm Paul, who pointedly observes that his prices are lower than in Beverly Hills. "It's half of a new Hyundai, but you probably get more mileage."

Paul reports few dissatisfied customers after more than a thousand such operations: "Today's the start of my seventeenth year here and I know I've never gone back and made them smaller."

Breast enhancement has been an emerging art for at least four decades. In the late 50s, the Japanese were injecting silicone, and some primitive implants secured with velcro were being used. But as a mass commercial phenomenon, enhancement most likely began back in 1964 with Carol Doda and her soon-famous 44 inch double D's.

Twenty silicone shots directly into the breasts of the San Francisco topless dancer turned a 24-year old well-proportioned cocktail waitress into a much publicized spectacle soon emulated throughout the world. The event was generally treated in the media as great fun, but the dancer had been exposed to what experts even then knew to be a dangerous procedure and one that is now illegal.

Current techniques employ sacs to keep the silicone gel from migrating throughout the body in disruptive ways, and the practice has moved from the realm of the bizarre to the respectable. In the booming cosmetic surgery trade, no procedure is more lucrative or controversial than breast augmentation.

Are modern breast enhancement procedures safe or dangerous? All experts agree that they should be described as major surgery, that anesthesia is required, and that, as with any such operation, serious complications and even death can occur.

This can happen even with highly trained, board-certified plastic surgeons, as with the case of another prominent Newport Beach doctor, currently under review by the state attorney general at the request of the Medical Board of California. In that case, the patient, a 35 year-old mother of four, was discovered unconscious in the recovery room of the doctor's office after routine breast augmentation surgery. She was taken by ambulance to a nearby hospital and died four days later. Family members charged that she had been deprived of oxygen and improperly monitored.

There have been other fatalities, but exact numbers are difficult to obtain because California, like most states, does not maintain statistics on deaths related to medical procedures. Local coroners will be informed, but they do not pass on the data, and in any case tend to report the cause of death as cardiac arrest without indicating whether it happened in the course of cosmetic surgery.

Responsible physicians routinely warn patients of the risks. There is, however, no common agreement on which procedures and implants are safest, and the patient is most often left wandering through a maze of competing claims in slick commercial advertisements. The choices, as bewildering as they are serious, were summarized by Dr. Lawrence N. Seifert, a leading Los Angeles surgeon:

"The patient and the surgeon have the option for three

locations of an incision: the armpit, the nipple, and underneath the breast; two locations of the implant: behind the muscle or above it; and five or six types of implants. You have 25 or 30 choices. Every one of these decisions has its own set of advantages and disadvantages and they need to be weighed on the scale of decision making."

Seifert, a spokesman for the American Society for Aesthetic Plastic Surgery, has performed this and other cosmetic procedures for more than 20 years. He says today's implants are safer and the techniques better than ever before, but acknowledges that the patient will often be at a loss to make difficult choices among competing medical claims.

One thing is clear: during the past 20 years, as women made choices about breast augmentation, regulatory authorities—state and federal—did nothing to provide them with impartial information about safe and wise procedures. They could not turn to the government for reliable information about which implants to use, the method of insertion and the location in the breast area, each of which are fraught with serious medical implications.

To date, most public attention has been paid to the risks associated with the implants themselves and they have recently been the subject of much media attention and Food and Drug Administration review.

Although two million American women have them, and American medical technology has made them common throughout the world, no one seems to know for sure whether these squiggly bags of silicone (or, less commonly, saline solution) are harmful inside the body and, if they are, just why.

The FDA, in effect, ignored the matter for 12 years until it ordered a comprehensive safety review in 1988 under pressure from congressional critics and patients' rights groups. In April of 1992, the agency ordered the manufacturers to supply proof of their products' safety.

It was only in September that the FDA, through Commissioner David A. Kessler, finally issued a serious warning: "Women need to be urged strongly to consider the risks of these implants . . . the implants have been on the market a long time and women have been lulled into thinking they are risk-free. They are not."

When the agency finally got around to requiring the manufacturers to document the safety of their implants, one leading company, Bristol-Myers Squibb, closed down its implant line instead. It advised doctors to cease using its polyurethane implant, which has been linked to carcinogens in some laboratory studies.

The FDA basically delayed a final decision on silicone implants. For the time being they may only be put in where needed for medical or reconstructive reasons. Those procedures will be monitored and after some unspecified time interval the FDA will decide whether to make the implants available once again to the general public. Non-silicone implants are of course still available and increasingly physicians have been using the ones that contain saline solution. If the bag should leak, saline is easily absorbed by the body and there should be no adverse health problems from a rupture of the implant.

In the meantime, there has been much lobbying for and against silicone implants, both before Congress and in the media. Critics of the implants have marshalled a list of patients to describe the dreadful consequences to their health which they attribute to silicone leaking and spreading to other parts of the body.

They argue that, as a result, some patients have experienced excruciating pain from cancer or autoimmune disease. Implant manufacturers and surgeons who specialize in breast enhancement have struck back with claims that the negative anecdotal evidence represents a statistically small proportion of implants and that the supposed consequences can often be attributed to other factors.

Recently, the controversy reached crescendo proportions. During hearings before the FDA in Washington in November of

1991, seven women testified about the painful consequences to their health of leaking silicone. Media accounts stressed their stories, but tended to overlook the upbeat endorsement provided by 44 other women who had received implants, some after mastectomies, and who called them important to their self-esteem. The arguments of some medical experts that the implants had not been properly tested were countered by a larger group of doctors and drug company representatives who contend that they are besieged by an irrational campaign mounted by know-nothings abetted by excessively litigious lawyers. Current odds lean toward the FDA simply requiring the manufacturers to collect more data, but the matter may be resolved in the courts.

Court cases are piling up on behalf of women who claim they have suffered dire consequences from the breast augmentation procedure. A recent article in a leading trial lawyers' magazine speaks of "an estimated 40% complication rate" and suggests that women who have received the implants may have much to talk to lawyers about.

Surgeons who perform the procedure, and many other medical experts, consider such charges absurd. They argue that the implants are safer than ever, that the complications refer mostly to the hardening resulting from the natural formation of scar tissue around the implant, which may be painful but is not generally medically threatening, and that true health risks are extremely low.

The safety of the silicone implants, while highly publicized, is not the only serious issue, as is made clear by the necessity to sift through competing claims about where to cut into the body and the best site for resting the implant. Because the FDA is authorized only to evaluate the safety of the implants themselves, questions of proper medical procedures or the qualifications of surgeons are not regulated. Decisions are left to the consultation between patient and doctor, and government, prodded by the well-organized medical lobby, has been loath to intervene. Yet those issues go directly to the question of comfort and safety.

"It's not a perfect operation. The patient should hear that loud and clear," says Seifert.

Of the three possible incision points (under the arm, the fold at the bottom of the breast, and the nipple), the nipple incision effectively hides the scar, but necessitates getting a rather large object through a small opening.

Most surgeons still prefer the fold incision since it provides the easiest and most visible access to the area where the implant will be placed. But it also leaves the most visible scar.

Dr. Thomas Stephenson, the West Los Angeles surgeon, champions the incision through the armpit.

"I've done over 3,000 and I feel good doing them," he said. He prefers it because unless the arms are raised, the scar will not be noticed, although it tends to be a bigger scar than in the other two locations.

His frequently placed ads in *The Los Angeles Times* headlined, "Every breast enhancement we perform is missing something," referring to the scar, are criticized by other surgeons who feel that he is ignoring the trade-off. In the underarm technique, the surgeon's vision is quite limited, they contend, though Stephenson disagrees, arguing that he has performed thousands satisfactorily.

"It's a blind dissection," says Seifert who has stopped using the procedure because "the surgeon really can't see exactly where he's doing it. In my practice, for about a year and a half, we did many of them and saw a significant complication range . . . The implant would end up at too high a level or they'd be different on both sides."

Seifert and other surgeons have said that placing the implant under the muscle allows it to be massaged constantly by the muscle's movement, mitigating the hardening or "encapsulation," which is the natural effort of the body to enclose, and protect itself against, a foreign object. This hardening, which occurs noticeably in an estimated 40% of implants above the muscle, can be quite unaesthetic and painful, necessitating surgical removal.

Paul, the Irvine surgeon, who claims 1,000 breast implants, is a fervent believer in the under-the-muscle technique and reports that with over-the-muscle implants, "40-60% of the breasts got firm. . . . We used to see a lot of those breasts that were pushed up and had the scar around them and that was obvious, but with the softer breasts now, the implants beneath the muscle and with the textured implants it's different. . . . Over 90% under the muscle stay soft. Years later they're still like butter."

A rougher or textured surface on the implants is known to mitigate the formation of scar tissue. Good results were reported with polyurethane coating, but there was suspicion that the coating itself might be carcinogenic. Currently, texture is provided by a rippling effect on the silicone surface of the implant sac. Hardening is down but there are complaints that the texturing causes a noticeable rippling of the skin itself.

The under-the-muscle technique is not generally considered effective for patients experiencing sagging of the breasts. Aesthetically you cannot attain as much projection of the breast as with the over-the-muscle implant. Also some doctors claim that with the under-the-muscle technique when a women flexes her muscles it can squeeze the implant and push it up or towards the side. Despite these drawbacks, statistics provided by the professional societies indicate that about 70% of doctors are now using the under-the-muscle procedure, but the controversy is not fully resolved.

In most doctors' offices, there are thick scrapbooks illustrating the negative effects of procedures rejected by that particular doctor and beneficial ones flowing from his chosen method. All one knows for sure is that the failed procedures can look grotesque, as is evidenced in the photos doctors routinely show patients to illustrate the negative consequences of alternative procedures.

What is a patient to do when starkly different views are offered by highly trained professionals arguing the merits of their own approach? The most common advice is, "Check with friends who have had the operation." But that may not be enough, because trouble may show up only much later.

One Newport Beach surgeon mentioned a recent case in which a woman who had breast implants placed by another doctor nine years ago came to see him. One of her breasts had suddenly hardened and she was in considerable pain. His best explanation is that this might have been triggered by an infection caused by a severe bout of the common cold.

As a precaution against hardening, this surgeon recommends an exercise to all of his implant patients, which involves lying on the abdomen for 15 minutes and vigorously moving the arms. He also suggests using a device called "Sta-sof(CQ)," widely advertised in the cosmetic literature. According to its inventor, Valerie Reid, it is "a clamp that goes behind the breast and compresses it to give continuous and consistent stretch pressure." She developed the device, she said, because "I would see women trying to massage their breasts with long nails, and they didn't have the necessary strength in their hands to stretch out the scar," which forms around the implant.

A federal epidemiologist, who has advised on congressional investigations and who asked that her name not be used, is skeptical of the claims of progress in dealing with the complications arising from breast augmentation. She observes that every few years a new technique is developed which is said to deal with the problems of the old one and then that method engenders its own complications and so some other method is found.

And there have also been a series of successful lawsuits against implant manufacturers. In December 1991, a federal court jury in San Francisco ordered Dow Corning to pay $7.34 million to a woman whose silicone breast implant ruptured, causing a painful disease of the immune system. The case is on appeal, and the company denies that there is any evidence linking the disease to the implant.

After years of steady growth, the market for breast implants has been hard hit by such unfavorable media reports and the economic recession. "I would say that business went down 25% or more—in some places, a lot more," reports Irvine's Paul. "New York City is a very depressed market now. But, it comes back as the economy rebounds. It's discretionary income. It's a new car, a family vacation, or a set of breast implants. It always follows that way, same as the car market, or the jewelry market."

Paul is not being frivolous, but as with other serious and professional surgeons, an inevitable commercialism creeps into his discussions about a procedure that involves purchasing breasts as a status symbol.

Nowhere is this more true than in Southern California. "We are a culture that is very much breast-oriented," Paul observes, "That's why it's very popular here. If you go to the beach and everyone else is filling a 'C' cup bathing suit and you're filling an 'A' cup, I don't think it would be unusual to feel self-conscious."

This socially induced feeling of being self-consciously inadequate is clearly basic to the rampant growth of the field of cosmetic surgery for both women and men. But while critics may bemoan such a mechanical measure of meaning and beauty in life, it remains a painful reality for those who, in increasing numbers, are choosing to undergo surgical procedures that carry serious risks.

As for Sue, who eight years after her operation wants C's instead of the B's her surgeon gave her, the choice is real, if depressing.

"Our society places so much value on the female figure that health issues take a back seat to fulfilling the fantasy and being accepted," she said. "Ideally, we should change the way that society views and values women."

But in the less than ideal world that she inhabits, she resents being told not to have the implants and views it as very much as a matter of personal choice whether "I forge ahead with a keen mind and a flat chest, or succumb to the pressures of society and buy a set of breasts like new silverware."

But it isn't like new silverware—it's your body and your health. And no matter the pressure to undertake any of the cosmetic surgery procedures, one ought to resist the quick decision and the blandishments of the more sales-oriented surgeons. All of the procedures involve similar points of controversy, differences of approach, and all present the same credentialing problems in selecting a surgeon as the breast implant procedure.

The difference, as I pointed out earlier, is not that breast implant procedures were more dangerous than liposuction, tummy-tucks or face lifts. On the contrary, the latter two are more dangerous procedures. Breast implants came to be regulated only because, as I said earlier, the implant itself is a medical product that is regulated by the FDA. There is no similar strenuous regulation of the doctors, their procedures and office setting. Sadly enough, as the articles in this book attest, the consumer/patient will be pretty much on his or her own in finding a safe procedure and a safe doctor.

The consumer may feel alone in his or her process of finding the appropriate doctor, appropriate procedure, or appropriate surgical facility. The consumer may also feel very confused. However, there is no need to be uninformed.

In the next section, we have compiled articles and testimony, descriptions and references. Once you have read through this material, you will know as much as anyone about procedures, current research, facts, and opinions. We have taken care to represent both sides of the certification question. We have attempted to be sensitive as well as candid about the risks. Our intention is that when you finish this book, you will have sufficient information to make the best decision for yourself, or at least know what questions to ask.

You may find yourself better-informed than some professionals.

THE TURF WAR

INTRODUCTION

Julius Newman, MD, before the House Committee on Small Businesses: *In 1979, a group of cosmetic surgeons decided there was the need for a new specialty, namely cosmetic surgery. Because this new specialty was so complex, and because there were so many new cosmetic surgical procedures, our group was convinced that this specialty had to be established as a separate discipline . . . Our position is that board certification in plastic and reconstructive surgery does not necessarily mean that the doctors are experienced and competent in cosmetic surgery.*

There is no group of doctors in any one specialty that have all the answers to perfect medical services, nor are all the finest surgeons in any one group. There are all levels of quality in our organization, as is true for the general plastic surgeons' organization.

       *   *   *

Lawrence Seifert, MD: *Good aesthetic surgery can be very rewarding and it can be very difficult to do. It's not something easy to learn. It takes years to be an accomplished aesthetic surgeon.*

I feel [the two-year residency represents] the first rungs on the ladder, and I think that the value of an approved residency in plastic and reconstructive surgery is that it teaches the surgeon a way to think. It gives the surgeon a set of basic principles upon which to build. And the building is a lifetime process that you must continue to pursue, as a violin virtuoso continues practicing, because complacency is the beginning of intellectual death . . . I'm happy to say that I really believe that the preponderance of my colleagues who I see year after year in medical meetings, scratching notes and drawing pictures, share this feeling with me. One of the great joys of being a plastic surgeon and being a member of an elite peer group is that you test each other, stimulate one another to do your best; you're critical of others' work, you're most critical of yourself; and I think that's a common denominator among the real plastic surgeons - the good plastic surgeons. You'd like to believe your doctor feels that way, wouldn't you?

* * *

What's the difference between a plastic surgeon and a cosmetic surgeon? Who is better qualified to perform elective, ɔurely aesthetic procedures? Are the two appellations even mutually exclusive?

The American Medical Association has no official policy or statement regarding plastic surgeons versus cosmetic surgeons. When asked about "board certification," representatives of the AMA offer to send a list of boards recognized by the AMA and which are identical to the member boards recognized by the American Board of Medical Specialties. These boards do not include the American Board of Cosmetic Surgery.

However, when asked specifically about cosmetic surgeons, a representative of the AMA will say that there are no official policies on cosmetic surgery as it is an "accepted medical practice."

So what's the fuss? Or did you even know there was a fuss?

Several issues are involved in what has been an extremely volatile, acrimonious debate. The surface issue involves certification of doctors performing surgery purely for cosmetic and aesthetic reasons. This type of surgery, by definition, is always elective and extremely lucrative—cash in advance. It's a tempting field for the MD, and the competition for a piece of the gold mine is cutthroat.

Surgeons trained and certified in plastic and reconstructive procedures claim that they are the only doctors qualified to perform such surgery. They say patients seeking a cosmetic surgeon should only look within the ranks of *board-certified* plastic and reconstructive surgeons. That is, certified by the American Board of Plastic Surgery which is recognized by the American Board of Medical Specialties which is recognized by the AMA, who will tell you that "cosmetic" surgery is also an accepted medical practice.

Where does *that* leave an inquiring consumer?

On the other hand, cosmetic surgeons, many of whom are ear, nose, and throat doctors who *do* have training in facial surgery, contend that a two-year residency in plastic and reconstructive surgery ill prepares a surgeon for cosmetic procedures, since the bulk of those two years is spent learning reconstructive procedures such as the reattachment of limbs, burns, and congenital deformities.

Most cosmetic surgeons, furthermore, *are* "board-certified" by the American Board of Medical Specialties in their respective specialty. In a few states, including California (Senate Bill 2036), "board-certified" has come by law to mean certification by the American Board of Plastic Surgery or a board with equivalent requirements. No cosmetic surgeon can claim board certification without meeting that restriction, or identifying the specialty in which he or she is certified. The specific languaging of the term "equivalent" is currently under debate, but has not yet been established.

Cosmetic surgeons claim that this law makes it difficult for them to compete; that in an advertisement for cosmetic surgery, the inability to claim board certification acts as a detriment to their business, becoming in effect a restraint of trade. For example, claiming board certification in gynecology could make a physician less attractive to a consumer seeking breast augmentation.

But there are members of the cosmetic group who have little or no surgical training, who attend a seminar or two, buy a fancy machine, and set themselves up as cosmetic "surgeons." Should this be allowed? How can a consumer tell whether such a physician is really qualified to do a good job on the desired procedure? The average consumer can't.

Another issue is advertising, traditionally frowned upon by the medical establishment and until a few years ago disallowed by the Federal Trade Commission. Doctors from both groups take advantage of the deregulation of advertising by the learned professions. In a society bombarded by and desensitized to advertising, the slicker the ad, the more attention is given to the product. We can not assume, however, that a doctor's capabilities can be judged by the attractiveness of his or her advertisement (we can only assess the talent of the art director). Unfortunately, most people do respond to advertising without considering the sales aspect. The success of the field of advertising

s directly proportional to its ability to manipulate. Many intelligent cosmetic surgery consumers respond to advertising, sometimes to their eternal chagrin.

Dr. John Reinisch, MD: *A lot of doctors are trying to sell
patients and capture them; for many doctors it's a business and
they're in it to make money. They've ceased to be as much of a
physician/doctor/counselor as a beautician who wants to make
the money and close the deal and pay their rent. When your
prime focus is making money, paying the rent, you're less likely
to be honest with a patient. That doesn't mean that they're
dishonest; it's just that they may be kidding themselves that they
can get a good result. [When] you have to pay the rent and you
haven't had a facelift in two months and it appears—a lady
walks in and that's a quick $6,000—it's very hard to say frankly,
"I don't think you're going to get your money's worth here."*

Since cosmetic surgery procedures are generally performed
in outpatient clinics, the issue of regulation becomes crucial. At
this writing, there is no regulation whatsoever. A researcher
hears many stories about plastic and cosmetic surgeons alike.
Eyewitnesses have seen sinks piled with dirty instruments,
waste receptacles overflowing with the previous day's bloody
towels, unlicensed technicians who may or may not know what
they're doing (in one case, it was the physician's young,
completely untrained niece). In one case, excised body parts
were kept in the freezer for future use in cosmetic surgery
cases, which are not covered by insurance, to send to labs as
dummy specimens, lending legitimacy to insurance claims. The
consumer, accustomed to being able to trust the doctor, finds
him- or herself in a position of having to check every detail,
including the adequacy of the surgical facility and their own
records for fraudulent insurance claims.

We consumers aren't trained to assess facilities or credentials,
or training, or expertise. Why should we be expected to? We
have been conditioned to trust our doctors simply because they
are doctors. We must bear in mind that surgeons are not gods,
but fallible human beings who get tired, hungry, and even

greedy, and who are capable of making mistakes. In considering cosmetic surgery, we are not shopping for a cosmetic product, nor even taking a chance like changing the cut or color of our hair. We are risking permanent disfigurement or even death by putting ourselves in the hands of a surgeon. And there is no way to figure the odds on any one particular surgeon, because there are no regulated standards. It seems like a roll of the dice.

The following articles illustrate this as yet unresolved conflict.

THE AMERICAN SOCIETY FOR AESTHETIC PLASTIC SURGERY
A Look at its Origin, Status, and Future

by Thomas J. Baker, M.D.

Plastic and Reconstructive Surgery
November 1982

[Editor's note: This article provides the most sensible solutions to the so-called "turf wars." Implementation of Dr. Baker's suggestions would greatly enhance public safty, patient care, and consumer satisfaction. Written ten years ago, his wise observations appear to have been ignored—KO]

Sal Castanares, in his Presidential Address in 1972, told us, "We cannot ignore the fact that the public has to expect every plastic surgeon to be competent in aesthetic surgery." . . . It has been estimated that 40 percent of the work done by plastic and reconstructive surgeons is aesthetic in nature, and it is quite probable that as much as 80 percent of plastic surgeons' incomes are derived from aesthetic surgery. . . . When a young plastic and reconstructive surgeon hangs a sign on his door that says, "Plastic Surgeon," the public believes that that individual is well-trained, especially in aesthetic surgery. But alas, such is not the case. . . . In my opinion, the trained aesthetic surgeon needs more than a "standard residency." . . . We cannot afford dilution with mediocrity!

. . . Our success is not measured by how many operations we do, but by how well we do them. It is apparent that the field of aesthetic surgery needs a suitable barometer by which to measure the qualifications and capabilities of those individuals doing aesthetic surgery, not only in our field, but in other branches of medicine who do some forms of aesthetic surgery. While we do have a barometer within our society, that is, Board Certification by the American Board of Plastic Surgery, it is quite possible that the day may come when the public, the government, or organized medicine itself may demand some type of certification in aesthetic surgery per se. The ability to do aesthetic surgery is difficult to judge by our current standards of examination as administered by the American Board of Plastic Surgery.

. . .

Many plastic surgeons are concerned that our "territory" of aesthetic surgery is being invaded by others. Is it really our territory? Do we really have one to call our own? We in plastic and reconstructive surgery formed a specialty taking a little bit from many other surgical specialties. We took from orthopedics, otolaryngology, dermatology, general surgery, ophthalmology, and so forth. Thus did we establish parameters for our specialty, but they are not absolute, and indeed, we do overlap into other "territories." There is much talk about inroads being made into our territory, especially from otolaryngology, dermatology, and ophthalmology. That this is happening is a fact . . . Can we look at [the] members of other specialties and say, "This is our territory and no one has the right to invade?" Certainly not. The fact that other specialties are going to be doing aesthetic surgery from this point forward is well known to all of us. I can foresee the day when there may be . . . an amalgamation of the various organizations doing aesthetic surgery in order to establish proper guidelines or to issue some type of certificate of competency. If this could be worked out, then all hospitals, state societies, clinics, and so forth would have a method to decide who in their community and in their respective areas are qualified to do aesthetic surgery. This problem must be faced. We cannot continue to ignore hundreds of other physicians outside of our own organization who are doing aesthetic surgery and just hope they will go away. . . . There are leaders in the various plastic surgery societies who seem to have tunnel vision and rarely look beyond our specialty. A wealth of information from our colleagues in other specialties is available to us if we but ask for it and share our experiences with them. We can learn much from others, but it will require a different type of cooperation than we have had in recent years. Why are we so concerned that our "territory" of aesthetic surgery is being invaded by others? Isn't it really economic more than any other one factor?

. . . It seems that we have already lost a legal (and moral) effort to restrict ourselves—meaning physicians engaged in aesthetic surgery—from advertising and utilizing the media for self-aggrandizement. . . . While advertising is distasteful to most of us, there doesn't seem to be a great deal we can do about the activity of others. . . . We must try to heal the wounds that exist between specialties or they will smolder and erode our very foundations. There really is a great deal to be gained by an exchange of information with these other specialty groups. . . . isolation is not the answer. If we stick our heads in the sand, we expose a much more vulnerable portion of our anatomy! We are not the only ones wearing white hats, and certainly all of our colleagues from other specialties do not all wear black hats. . . .

We who have reached the position in our profession that we now enjoy are here because we stood on the shoulders of those who preceded us. By continuing to set the standards of excellence in this society through research, adequate training, and continued exchange of scientific information, the membership of the American Society for Aesthetic Plastic Surgery can provide those who succeed us even stronger shoulders on which to stand.

To repeat, we cannot afford dilution with mediocrity.

SPECIALTIES FEUD OVER COSMETIC SURGERY AT HEARING

By Flora Johnson Skelly

American Medical News

April 28, 1989

Like a family argument that erupts into a shouting match in a grocery store, a simmering feud between specialty groups turned public and acrimonious during recent congressional hearings on cosmetic surgery. Testimony before the . . . House Committee on Small Business pitted two specialty groups against a third as members of Congress, reporters, and TV cameras looked on.

At the center of the debate was a burgeoning new field of medical care—cosmetic surgery, medicine's answer to man's physical imperfections. Demand for procedures such as "tummy tucks," liposuction, and breast implants is growing, fueled by advertising that often seems to promise beauty without risk. Medical practitioners from various specialties are meeting this demand, and therein lies the controversy. . . .

At issue: Which group or groups of specialists are qualified to perform cosmetic surgery?

On one side was the American Society of Plastic and Reconstructive Surgeons Inc. (ASPRS), which represents approximately 3,000 physicians certified by the American Board of Plastic Surgery Inc. This board has been recognized as an independent specialty by the American Board of Medical Specialties (ABMS) and the AMA since 1941.

The board certifies physicians after they've earned their medical degrees, completed at least three years of approved training in general surgery or been certified in otolaryngology or orthopedic surgery, finished an accredited two- to three-year residency program in plastic surgery, passed a written qualifying examination, practiced the specialty for two years, passed an oral exam, and been reviewed for professional and ethical fitness. Subsequently the physician must meet standards in continuing medical education to remain board-certified.

To become a member of the ASPRS a physician must meet additional requirements, including adherence to a code of ethics that forbids false, fraudulent, or deceptive advertising.

"There is a growing number of physicians and surgeons whose greed outweighs ethics and concern for patient well-being," Dr. [Norman] Cole [of the ASPRS] said. "They either refuse to accept the decision of their peers or avoid the peer review process altogether, realizing that they do not possess the training or experience to qualify for hospital privileges. Instead, they establish unlicensed and unaccredited surgical facilities in their offices, or build surgical clinics, and aggressively market themselves and their facilities to an unsuspecting public."

. . . Other specialties involved in cosmetic surgery, however, contend that the plastic surgeons are exploiting or even exaggerating these problems as part of a campaign to persuade consumers that only board-certified plastic surgeons are qualified to perform cosmetic surgery. Quality of care is not the issue in this debate, they say: rather, this is a "turf war" in which the plastic surgeons are attempting to keep other, equally qualified specialties out of a lucrative and growing market.

One of these groups is the American Board of Cosmetic Surgery, which represents some 250 physicians who say they have created a new specialty called "cosmetic surgery." The specialty was needed because cosmetic surgery had become "so complex" and "there were many new cosmetic surgical

procedures, along with there being an unexpected high demand by the general public for cosmetic surgery," Julius Newman,
MD, president of the cosmetic surgery board, told the subcommittee. The board, created by approximately 150 cosmetic surgeons who were "grandfathered" into the organization, held its
first board exam in 1982.

Candidates for full certification by the cosmetic surgery board
must now be certified in otolaryngology surgery, general surgery,
plastic and reconstructive surgery, gynecology, dermatology, or
maxillofacial surgery. Those certified in maxillofacial surgery
must have MD and DDS degrees. The maxillofacial surgeons
and dermatologists also must take a year of general surgery.

In addition, the candidate for full certification in cosmetic
surgery must follow one of two paths: He may complete an
approved one-year fellowship and demonstrate that he has
performed 500 cosmetic surgical procedures since finishing his
fellowship program, or he may demonstrate that he has performed 1,000 cosmetic surgical procedures within the last five
years. (At least 200 procedures must have been performed
within the last year.) Having been evaluated on character and
background, the candidate then sits for a written exam, followed
by an oral exam. Currently, Dr. Newman said, approximately
60% of those who take these exams pass them.

The cosmetic surgery board contends that its certification
procedures are comparable to those applied by the board of
plastic surgeons. Indeed, these physicians contend, plastic surgery is such a large field that, during his residency in plastic and
reconstructive surgery, a surgeon devotes only a portion of his
time to cosmetic surgical techniques. Thus, Dr. Newman told
the subcommittee, "board certification in plastic and reconstructive surgery does not necessarily mean that the doctors are
experienced and competent in cosmetic surgery."

The plastic surgeons' response to this contention is vitriolic.
They point out first that the cosmetic surgery board has not
been recognized by the ABMS and AMA. (It is unlikely cosmetic
surgery would be recognized as an independent specialty, be-

cause ABMS policy rules out recognizing more than one specialty per field.) Second, the plastic surgeons say that the cosmetic surgery board does not require residency training in "a field related to cosmetic surgery" before it will certify someone in cosmetic surgery. Finally, they protest that the existence of this board, and of physicians who call themselves "board certified" after meeting its criteria, creates confusion among consumers who may erroneously believe that all board certification is alike.

To the ASPRS criticisms, the cosmetic surgery board responds that it is a new group, and has not had enough time to become fully established yet. "No board that was ever established was able to begin in totally satisfactory academic and practical fashion," Dr. Newman said.

Another organization involved in the dispute with the plastic surgeons is the American Academy of Facial Plastic and Reconstructive Surgery, a constituent specialty of the AMA and American College of Surgeons consisting of more than 3,000 surgeons from various specialties involved in cosmetic and reconstructive surgery of the head and neck. These include plastic surgeons, ophthalmologists, and dermatologists, but the vast majority are otolaryngologists. Members of this academy must be board-certified in an ABMS-recognized specialty, be fellows of the college of surgeons, and demonstrate competence in facial plastic surgery.

This group took a strong stand in favor of diversity among the specialties involved in cosmetic surgery, arguing in a statement submitted to the subcommittee that "recognition of skilled surgeons from various specialties benefits the consumer." The statement went on to deny that "there is any special problem of incompetence in facial plastic surgery. . . . The academy is aware of no evidence that facial plastic surgery has any larger percentage of less skilled practitioners than any other field."

At the hearings, the facial plastic surgeons joined the cosmetic surgeons in accusing plastic surgeons of unfair trade practices. They complained bitterly about advertisements such as ones they displayed at the hearing, which was sponsored by the Dallas Society of Plastic Surgeons. Headlined "Not everyone who does plastic surgery is a plastic surgeon," it states, "Not all doctors who perform plastic surgery are plastic surgeons. The fact is, some doctors are only taking quick courses to learn cosmetic procedures. However, you can trust doctors certified by the American Board of Plastic Surgery. They have gone through years of training in plastic surgery of the face and body. . . . Choose an expert who's fully trained as a plastic surgeon." The facial plastic surgeons contend that such ads imply plastic surgery can be performed only or best by those whom the facial plastic surgeons refer to as "general plastic surgeons."

. . . At the hearing, Dr. [John R.] Jarrett [of the ASPRS] stated that some specialists other than plastic surgeons are qualified to do specific cosmetic surgery procedures for which they are trained in residency, and specifically mentioned that plastic surgeons have "no argument" with otolaryngologists performing cosmetic surgery of the head and neck. Plastic surgeons are concerned only, he said, that some physicians are doing procedures not within their specialty. "Physicians whose formal training is limited to otolaryngology—or dermatology, gynecology, family practice, etc.—*are* advertising their willingness to perform breast augmentation and body sculpturing—often attached to a claim of board certification and the self-designated title of 'cosmetic surgeon,'" Dr. Jarrett said. . . .

The cosmetic surgeons and facial plastic surgeons, however, expressed concern that any attempt to regulate advertising would be used as a vehicle to exclude specialties other than plastic surgery from the field of cosmetic surgery.

In an interview, Dr. Newman stated that cosmetic surgeons agree there is a need to regulate advertising in the field of cosmetic surgery, but that such regulations must affect all specialties equally. Cosmetic surgeons would prefer that regulation come from within the medical community rather than from government, however, Dr. Newman said.

The cosmetic surgery board would accept a requirement

that advertisers state what board certified them, he said. But the cosmetic surgeons would resist an attempt to insist that they state that their board is not recognized by the ABMS, or other restrictions that, they believe, would favor the plastic surgeons. Speaking for the American Academy of Facial Plastic and Reconstructive Surgery, board member and past president Robert L. Simons, MD, said his organization "does not believe there is any special problem of deceptive advertising in facial plastic surgery." Complaints about unethical advertising "come, by and large, from entrenched incumbent surgeons unhappy about new competitors," Dr. Simons said.

Another issue evidently important to Wyden was regulation of ambulatory care facilities. In his introductory remarks, he said that . . . cosmetic surgery procedures are being done in physicians' offices, "outside of hospitals and the protective eye of surgical review boards. Coast to coast, these office practices are touted as 'institutes,' 'centers,' and 'clinics' of cosmetic surgery in the more expansive ads. In too many cases, we see one doctor in a spartan surgical setting with a skeleton crew. Too often they lack the most basic life-support systems found in the smallest hospital emergency rooms. Neither are we sure that personnel with even the most rudimentary technical training assist in these procedures."

Listing ASPRS proposals, Dr. Jarrett told the House subcommittee that physicians should be permitted to perform cosmetic plastic surgery in their offices only if they have first received privileges to do the same procedures in an accredited hospital. In addition, all office surgical facilities should be approved by an outside, independent accrediting body, he said.

"Even if a practitioner intends to perform surgical procedures outside of the hospital setting, the public deserves the assurance that the physician does meet hospital standards," said Dr. Cole, who called peer review "the most meaningful assurance of quality control in plastic surgery."

. . . Acknowledging that "many office-based surgical facilities are not adequate," Dr. Newman announced that the cosmetic surgeons board has decided in 1990, before a physician whose surgery is entirely office-based can take the qualifying exam, he either will have to show that he has hospital surgical privileges or will have to be examined by two certified cosmetic surgeons who will evaluate his surgical facility, observe his surgery, review his record keeping, and evaluate his entire operation. The board is also instituting a program of peer review at five-year intervals, Dr. Newman said.

The ASPRS proposal that no physician should be allowed to do a procedure in his office that he is not credentialed to do in a hospital is a problem for cosmetic surgeons, however, because of their contention that they may be blocked from hospital privileges by prejudice against their new specialty. In an interview, Dr. Newman rejected the ASPRS proposal, saying that such a requirement would be a restraint of trade.

One of the overriding impressions left by the . . . testimony was that while the variety of practitioners involved in cosmetic surgery may well bring all the benefits of competition to this marketplace, consumers do, indeed, face daunting difficulties in sorting out which practitioners are best qualified to perform specific procedures.

"The consumer has a wide variety of choices," Wyden said in his closing remarks, "and what we've heard is that very often these choices are presented in such a way that consumers find it very difficult to determine who is a qualified practitioner and who isn't. . . . Consumers find it very difficult in my view to make the best and most appropriate choices for them. It's the chair's sense . . . that patients deserve more."

WHO IS QUALIFIED TO PERFORM COSMETIC SURGERY?

CONGRESSIONAL TESTIMONY

HOW TO SELECT A QUALIFIED PHYSICIAN
A Public Safety Issue

Presented by
Harvey Zarem, MD
Past Director and Senior Examiner
American Board of Plastic Surgery

Committee for Public Information on
Aesthetic Surgery Issues
American Society for Aesthetic Plastic Surgery

April 4, 1989
Subcommittee on Regulation, Business Opportunities
and Energy Committee on Small Business
U.S. House of Representatives

. . .

How *does* one go about finding a trained and competent plastic surgeon?

Articles in the lay press often instruct consumers to ask the physician direct questions aimed at discovering how much experience he or she has in a particular procedure, and to examine before and after photos of previous patients. These approaches may be helpful, to some extent, in determining the experience of the physician, and most plastic surgeons have many examples of their work to show prospective patients. However, it is common logic to assume that any doctor will show the best surgical results, not the worst. What still remains unknown to the patient is the depth of training which qualifies a particular doctor to perform the procedures in question; and it is depth of training alone which is the patient's best assurance of the doctor's ability to exercise appropriate judgment in any surgical situation, whether routine or dealing with unforeseeable complications.

Every human being has an intuitive sense, and patients should be encouraged to use their instincts when evaluating a doctor. If any physician does not provide honest, frank and thorough answers to questions posed by a prospective patient, this should be an important warning sign. If a physician does not voluntarily discuss both the benefits and risks of a surgical procedure, this should also be of concern to the patient. If a physician makes unrealistic statements or promises regarding the results of surgery, the patient should beware. However, the technical aspects of plastic surgery, or any medical specialty, are often difficult for the patient to understand and evaluate. In addition, a physician may be a very effective communicator, using a "slick" approach or various methods of persuasion which succeed in overcoming the patient's own better judgment. The qualified and honest physician will often appear less attractive to the patient when compared with this type of smooth-talking salesman. So, obviously, intuition is not enough when trying to select a qualified doctor.

Another avenue which is often suggested to patients seeking a qualified plastic surgeon is the recommendation of their family doctor. This can be a valid approach, but it, too, has major pitfalls. It has often occurred that a highly competent and conscientious physician has innocently referred a patient to a doctor known by his immediate colleagues to be disreputable. This is unlikely to occur if the referring doctor knows the other physician through a hospital or teaching institution affiliation which has required some form of credentialing and selective process. Nevertheless, it is surprising and sad to realize that many patients have fallen into the hands of unqualified doctors through the advice of a trusted physician.

The point of this discussion has been to show that the public is at significant risk when trying to select a qualified physician. The most reliable measure of competence remains appropriate education and certification by a medical specialty board approved by the American Board of Medical Specialties— in the case of plastic surgery, certification by the American Board of Plastic Surgery.

The problem for the consumer is to separate fact from fiction, lies from truth, and meaningful credentials from spurious ones. Since this is a responsibility for which most of the public is unprepared, it is up to society to protect individuals from possible serious consequences, both physical and psychological, by establishing appropriate regulations which curtail the ability of physicians to misrepresent their qualifications.

A PLASTIC SURGEON SPEAKS ON BEHALF OF COSMETIC SURGEONS

Statement of
Richard C. Webster, M.D.

On Behalf of the American Board of Cosmetic Surgery, and The American Academy of Cosmetic Surgery, before the House Committee of Regulation and Business Opportunities
April 4, 1989

I satisfied the requirements and passed the examinations necessary to become Board Certified in Plastic Surgery — some 35 years ago. Not one operation . . . in the much more specialized field of cosmetic surgery, did I learn during my required years enabling me to "get my Boards." Many of the procedures (liposuction, breast implants, etc.) had not even been invented. The actual techniques used in all the operations have changed totally or greatly with surgical progress. . . .

Still, that board certificate permitted me, as an expert or a specialist in the entire field of plastic surgery, to get on the staffs of many hospitals and "entitled" me . . . to have privileges to do essentially every procedure listed in the huge fields of plastic and maxillofacial surgery—limited *only* by my conscience and pride in doing well what I did do. . . . Just because organized medicine endorsed the system that makes this series of events possible does not make the system right. In fact, it does not protect the public properly in today's increasingly sophisticated and competitive world.

. . . Citizens in a society . . . must never relinquish their final say (through elected officials) in deciding just whom to license to provide them their health care. While many doctors genuinely believe, as I do, that they think always of the patient's good above their own, they *do* have a vested financial interest in providing that care. In spite of organized medicine's and dentistry's best efforts, there have been enough abuses to prove that never should final authority as to licensing be turned over to the providers. . . .

. . . The emergence of any new specialty is likely to be resisted by those who have competitively motivated desires to hold back the new and more specialized group. . . . In certain states, though I specialize only in cosmetic surgery, I would not be able to advertise as such. I *am* required to either say that I am a plastic surgeon (though I do none of the hundreds of plastic surgical procedures except for the small number of cosmetic operations), or where I am allowed to say that I am also board certified in cosmetic surgery, I *must then add* that my board certification in cosmetic surgery is not approved by organized medicine.

. . . And, as long as the organized plastic surgeons retain their present clout in organized medicine, the cosmetic surgical board *will not get approval.* I submit that cosmetic surgery is *now* a specialty and that the consuming public knows this to be true. . . .

Although I specialize . . . more than most plastic surgeons, I am effectively denied any right to tell the consumer just that. This anticompetitive result of the present system provided by organized medicine and dentistry must be eliminated. . . .

THE ABMS
PRESENTS ITS VIEW

Testimony of
Peyton E. Weary, M.D.
and Donald G. Langsley, M.D.

on behalf of The American Board of
Medical Specialties at the hearings on
Cosmetic Surgery

Presented to:
The Subcommittee on
Regulation and Business Opportunities of the
United States House of Representatives
June 28, 1989

. . . the statement that a physician is "board certified" is not
enough. There are at least 105 self-designated boards of which
we know and there is no system for guaranteeing that such
boards meet the high standards required for ABMS [American
Board of Medical Specialties] and AMA [American Medical
Association] approval and recognition. In our country, anyone
can organize a "board" and name it the "American Board of
whatever." Those who organize such boards set their own
standards. They may waive any required education and may
waive any examination process. A few of these self-designated
boards have high standards and require residency training plus
an examination in a fashion similar to that of the ABMS
member boards. We have encouraged them to consider appli-

cation for recognition and approval. Most, however, do not seem to meet such standards. Our knowledge of their organizations, sponsors and systems is often scanty, and in response to queries from various physicians, they only release brochures urging the respondent to apply and pay certain fees. In contrast, the organization, requirements and systems of the ABMS member boards are public knowledge.

This presents a serious dilemma to the American public which does not know the difference between certification by an ABMS-approved board and a self-designated board. To the average citizen the advertisement of being "board certified" carries with it an expected level of qualifications and competence which may not coincide with reality. If a physician is a member of the medical staff of a hospital accredited by the Joint Commission on the Accreditation of Health Care Organizations (JCAHO) and has privileges to practice in that hospital it generally indicates that the qualifications of the physician to claim board certification have been reviewed. However, many physicians confine their practice to their private offices or to unaccredited alternative sites. The average citizen who may have extensive and complex treatment, including surgery, in a private office could view the display of a "certificate" from a self-designated board or the advertisement of "board certified" as assurance of protection which is deceptive. We have tried to increase public awareness of this situation, but you will understand what a challenge it is to educate all of America about this complex process.

SELECTING A COSMETIC SURGEON: IT'S MORE THAN SKIN DEEP

By Richard Caleel, D.O., F.A.C.S.

The American Academy of Cosmetic Surgery, the largest organization representing physicians in the field of cosmetic surgery, warns prospective cosmetic surgery patients to be wary of surgeons who state their qualifications based only on board certification. In the case of some certifying bodies, board certification can simply mean minimal training and may not even require proof of on-going proficiency in a specialized area.

The American Academy of Cosmetic Surgery's certifying board has established a strict set of criteria to ensure safe and successful cosmetic procedures. A physician certified by this board must comply with the following:

1) Be board certified in an original discipline or specialty recognized by the American Board of Medical Specialties and the American Medical Association.

2) Have been in the practice (primarily) of cosmetic surgery for the last five years.

3) Have performed no less than 1,000 cosmetic operations.

4) Be currently performing no less than 200 documented cosmetic procedures per year.

5) Pass a stringent oral and written exam.

6) Be of good moral character.

Courtesy of American Academy of Cosmetic Surgery.

REQUIREMENTS FOR FULL CERTIFICATION AND AREAS OF CERTIFICATION AMERICAN BOARD OF COSMETIC SURGERY

Applicants for certification, whether full or partial, must have been performing surgery in their specialty for a minimum of five (5) years, and must have completed a minimum of one thousand (1,000) cosmetic surgical procedures, of which at least two hundred (200) have been performed within the twelve (12) month period immediately prior to application for certification.

Applicants for certification, whether full or partial, must successfully complete a written examination covering general knowledge of cosmetic surgical procedures.

Applicants for full certification must successfully complete an oral examination in each of the following categories:

1) Body & Extremity Cosmetic Surgery
2) Cosmetic Breast Surgery
3) Dermatologic Cosmetic Surgery
4) Facial Cosmetic Surgery

Applicants for partial certification must successfully complete an oral examination in each category for which certification is desired.

A credentials committee established by the president shall recommend for membership to the Board of Trustees those applicants who have satisfied the certification requirements.

1) Applicants for certification, whether full or partial, should be board certified in one of the following: American

Board of Medical Specialties (ABMS), American Osteo-
pathic Association (AOA) or equivalent specialties:
- Dermatology
- General Surgery
- Gynecology
- Maxillofacial Surgery (with dual M.D. and D.D.S.)
- Ophthalmology
- Orthopedics
- Otolaryngology/Head and Neck
- Plastic and Reconstructive

2) Applicants for certification, whether full or partial, must:

(a) submit letter of recommendation from the chairper-
son of his or her residency of other training program or from the department chief at his or her
current hospital facility; or

(b) if the applicant has no current hospital operating
room privileges and who performs all surgical procedures in his/her office, applicant must submit to a
visit and inspection by cosmetic surgeons selected
by the Board who will inspect the surgical facilities,
observe and evaluate live procedures and examine
patient records. The total cost of the inspection will
be borne by the applicant.

TRAINING IN THE SPECIALTY AREA OF FACIAL PLASTIC SURGERY VS. TRAINING IN PLASTIC SURGERY

FACIAL PLASTIC SURGEON	PLASTIC SURGEON
AAFPRS Fellowship in Facial Plastic Surgery 1 Year	
Residency in Otolaryngology/ Head and Neck Surgery, including facial plastic surgery 4 to 5 Years	Residency in Plastic Surgery 2 Years
General Surgery Residency 1 Year	General Surgery Residency 3 - 4 Years
Medical School 4 Years	Medical School 4 Years
College 4 Years	College 4 Years

FACIAL PLASTIC SURGEON   **PLASTIC SURGEON**

AMERICAN ACADEMY OF FACIAL PLASTIC AND RECONSTRUCTIVE SURGERY

AESTHETIC PLASTIC SURGERY PERSPECTIVES FROM A PRIVATE PRACTITIONER

by Larry Seifert, MD, FACS

The art of Plastic Surgery is to restore those parts which nature hath given and malfortune hath taken away, not all to delight the eye but buoy the spirits of the afflicted.

—Gaspar Tagalcozzi, 1597

The word plastic, as in aesthetic plastic surgery, is derived from the Greek *plastikos*, which means to mold or give form. The plastic surgeon seeks to mold and reshape contours of the human body. Aesthetic plastic surgery is performed to enhance a person's body or facial features. It is part of the unique specialty of plastic surgery which also includes reconstructive surgery. The latter restores form and function to disfigurements caused by trauma, disease, or birth defects. While aesthetic surgery is elective, it is nevertheless surgery. There is nothing superficial or trivial in the decision to have the operation, and the selection of a trained and qualified aesthetic plastic surgeon

[Dr. Seifert is an Assistant Clinical Professor at the UCLA School of Medicine Department of Plastic Surgery and the former Chairman of Plastic Surgery at Cedars-Sinai Medical Center in Los Angeles. A member of the American Society of Plastic and Reconstructive Surgery and the American Society of Aesthetic Plastic Surgery, he is currently in private practice in Beverly Hills, California - KO]

is the single most important factor in its success.

The psychological implications inherent in an aesthetic surgical change of body and facial image are profoundly complex and unique for each person. There is a strong motivation to look our personal best and present a positive image to the world. Poets and artists have paid homage to physical beauty since the time of antiquity. In today's world, the benefits of good aesthetic surgery are available to most of us—not just to movie stars and the very wealthy.

Every plastic and reconstructive surgeon performing aesthetic surgery knows of the joy and pleasure experienced by grateful patients when surgical results match preoperative expectations. Enhanced self-esteem and measurable social benefits can be achieved by aesthetic plastic surgery. In his 1977 Harvard University psychology doctorate, Dr. Kalick concluded that aesthetic plastic surgery increased self-awareness of physical attractiveness. In his study, women [who] benefited by aesthetic surgery were seen as kinder, more sensitive, more sexual and so forth.

However, realistic expectations are essential to achieving satisfaction through aesthetic plastic surgery. Even the most successful surgical outcome will not solve your personal problems and is no guarantee of happiness or improved interpersonal relationships. Moreover, each operation has its own specific risks and complications. No operation is *free of all risk*, just as nothing in life is completely "safe." It is the duty of the responsible aesthetic plastic surgeon to carefully evaluate the physical and psychological appropriateness of each potential candidate for aesthetic surgery. The surgeon must not only provide the patient with all available information on the benefits and risks of procedures, but must also help the patient put these facts into personal perspective. The aesthetic plastic surgeon is first a medical doctor, and second a surgeon with the ability to help patients achieve a more positive self-image.

These days not all physicians who perform cosmetic operations are fully or equally trained. In fact, there is no state or federal law prohibiting any licensed physician to proclaim themselves a self-designated expert in cosmetic surgery. Within the hospital environment, regulatory mechanisms by peer review determine surgical privileges to be performed in the operating room. The process of peer review is vital to ensure minimum standards for patient care. In the hospital, only a neurosurgeon performs brain surgery. Outside the safety net of hospital rules and regulations, the process of peer review is legally non-existent. Best estimates by the American Society of Plastic and Reconstructive Surgeons (ASPRS) indicate fully 80% of all aesthetic surgery is performed outside the hospital, in private surgical suites. Putting it in simpler terms, the coffee shop cheeseburgers in the very same medical building are inspected by the state, but no state agency inspects the outpatient operating rooms. This need to inspect and accreditate both staff and facility has been addressed by organized plastic surgery with the establishment of the American Association for Accreditation of Ambulatory Plastic Surgical Facilities (AAAAPSF), which inspects and accredits office-based surgical facilities. However, AAAAPSF accreditation is available only to plastic and reconstructive surgeons certified by the American Board of Plastic Surgery.

Certification by the American Board of Plastic Surgery (ABPS) is one prerequisite to membership in the nation's oldest and largest organization in plastic surgery, the American Board of Plastic and Reconstructive Surgery (ASPRS). The wide knowledge possessed by the fully trained, complete plastic and reconstructive surgeon, allows application of the basic principles to perfect the special skill necessary to be an excellent aesthetic surgeon. Some members of ASPRS pursue a special interest in aesthetic surgery and apply for membership in the American Society for Aesthetic Plastic Surgery (ASAPS). The Aesthetic Society (ASAPS) was founded in 1967 and is devoted to promoting advanced knowledge, research, and training in aesthetic surgery.

ASAPS has nearly 1000 members nationwide, all of whom

have:

1) Completed at least 3 years of private practice since certification by the American Board of Plastic Surgery.

2) As a candidate, were carefully reviewed by a select membership committee and approved for ASAPS membership by four-fifths of participating active members.

3) Devoted a significant portion of their plastic surgical practice to complex aesthetic operations.

Why all this training and education if the surgeon focuses in a narrow sphere? The complete aesthetic plastic surgeon is trained in an anatomic three dimensional sense. This surgeon sees the important inter-relationships of skin, fat, muscle, and bone. Today's increasingly complex and sophisticated operative techniques require this broad education. As in the arts, one must first master the basics in order to proceed with the finest artistic endeavors.

It has been argued in some quarters that surgical skills in reconstruction and aesthetic surgery are mutually exclusive. This position ignores the all-important relationship between form, function, and beauty. A UCLA plastic surgery conference in August, 1992, illustrates this point. The comprehensive three-hour meeting was devoted to facial aesthetic surgery: face and forehead lift. Moss Auditorium was filled to capacity with medical students, residents, and faculty. The darkened room was illuminated by twin slide projectors beaming before and after photographic images, which document our surgical results. The audience of plastic surgeons compared and contrasted the classic facelift with the newer deep plane rhytidectomy, an extended lift crossing the cheek bone, going to the side of the nose, and reaching the upper lip. Does the new technique achieve a maximum improvement in the mid third of the face? Upon the screens, the images showed loose skin becoming taut, revealing pleasing sculpted facial bone contours previously obscured by aging. Years melted away. This new rhytidectomy technique relies upon a basic reconstructive principle, the subcutaneous flap (skin plus deeper tissues), and is benefited by an enriched blood supply. This in turn favors better healing.

The principle of this composite flap was pioneered in reconstructive surgery over twenty years ago. It is utilized to repair deformities of limb, breast, and trunk and now is used in aesthetic plastic surgery as one of the newest techniques for facial rejuvenation.

The scientific session ended three hours after it had begun. Two of us left the auditorium and spoke sharing our opinions of the conference. The younger surgeon was finishing his eleventh year of medical training after four years of college; the older clinical faculty member had practiced for over twenty years. The younger surgeon's thoughts shifted from aesthetics to reconstruction as he spoke of microsurgical free flaps in breast reconstruction. There was a smooth transition of thought from aesthetic to reconstructive surgery.

There are no short cuts. An immense fund of knowledge is required in order to think and see. A unique combination of science and art bridges between beauty, form, and function. Years ago, when we were young surgical residents, my partner, Dr. E. W. Worton, looked to our future and said: "It's worth it in the long run."

ADVERTISING

BUYER BEWARE
A Memo to
Congressman
Ron Wyden

by Wyden Congressional Staff

Date: MARCH 27, 1989

To: CHAIRMAN RON WYDEN

From: SUBCOMMITTEE STAFF

Subject: UNQUALIFIED DOCTORS PERFORMING
           COSMETIC SURGERY: MUST THE "BUYER
           BEWARE" IN THIS MULTI-BILLION DOLLAR
           MEDICAL INDUSTRY?

Over the last several years, many patients of cosmetic surgery have been seriously injured and some have died following elective cosmetic procedures. It appears that the field is being overrun by less than fully qualified doctors operating with little or no oversight by either government or their peers. Fully 95 percent of all cosmetic surgery procedures are now done outside of hospitals, in doctors' offices or in limited service clinics.

Based on the staff's six-month investigation, it appears that the government has become an unwitting accomplice by making consistently uninformed and ill-conceived decisions on how to

guarantee safe, affordable medical care. The Federal Trade
Commission stands alone in having taken one dramatic—and
many say disastrous—step that has crippled the medical profession and left the American consumer virtually defenseless.

The FTC declared war on the learned professions as it
implemented the Federal Trade Commission Improvement Act
of 1975. . . .With its federal court victory over the AMA and two
Connecticut medical organizations, the FTC threw open the
regulatory door for medical advertising. Not only did it send the
message that the FTC would *not* prohibit the peddling of medicine, *it made it virtually impossible for the medical profession to
police its own to ensure ethical standards and quality care.*

This should come as no surprise to the FTC. The agency
actually *anticipated and accepted* that there would be serious
risks to patients. As one FTC staffer said,

> "I won't deny the fact that some people
> will go into brain surgery and have conse-
> quences that we all don't want. There will
> be costs—really serious costs—but the
> benefits are that we will know what the
> hell is going on in the medical market-
> place."

The FTC was right. We do know much more about the
medical marketplace. We know that most patients take at face
value cosmetic surgeons' ads. We know that they think most
cosmetic surgery is safe. We know that they think it's safe to
have surgery done in doctors' offices, not just in hospitals . . .
we know that the FTC's medical marketplace has become a
multi-billion dollar industry in the cosmetic surgery field alone.

Unfortunately, we also know that countless patients are
being injured. They are being physically and emotionally scarred
and they are being financially drained.

Even when potential patients try to be "good medical
consumers," they run into a stone wall erected by state and
federal governments, medical societies and individual doctors

themselves. With a lot of help from the FTC and some in the medical profession, it has become virtually impossible for patients to tell who is a good, qualified doctor and who is not.

And the marked trend toward outpatient surgery has removed the last vestige of accountability for many doctors. No hospital review board verifies the quality of these surgeons' work. No one guarantees whether the "operating room" has even basic life support equipment. No one ensures that the doctor has good, qualified staff to give anesthetic, to monitor the patient and to respond quickly should complications arise.

The frightening result may be that the new back alley of medicine has become the doctor's office itself. We have found that, incredibly, any doctor who manages to graduate from medical school, and receive a state license, can do anything, be anything. Anyone with a medical degree and a state license can do brain surgery, face lifts, breast reductions or enlargements—even open heart surgery.

This situation exists in every state in the country. But many believe such an environment is far from ethical. Competition has, indeed, come to the medical profession.

The staff has identified the following type of cosmetic surgery ads that should send a red warning flag up to the consumer *and* the FTC. Advertisements that:

— contain promises about the physical results of surgery;
— contain statements about the surgical procedure;
— contain claims about the innovative character of an operation;
— contain false claims about the physician or his or her staff;
— contain so-called "before and after" photographs, with the "after" photograph posed in a more favorable angle and lighting;
— show the results of one patient's experience or one person's testimonial to apparently imply and mislead other people to conclude that anyone having the same

operation *can and should* have a similar result;

— utilize truthful information in a manner that may mislead potential patients as to the qualifications of the advertising physician. An example is one physician who included his membership in the AMA as part of his qualifications. Membership in the AMA is *not* a function of professional skill;

— assert that a physician is qualified as a "board certified cosmetic surgeon" when no board of that title is recognized by the American Board of Medical Specialties;

— claim board certification when they are actually certified in other specialties having little or nothing to do with the cosmetic surgery procedures being performed;

— advertise credentials, perhaps impressive to lay persons but medically meaningless, including authorship of articles published in obscure medical journals;

— state doctor inventions of surgical instruments;

— state special residency training and expertise;

— claim state-of-the-art facilities and invite visits by patients who want to make comparisons. Most potential patients have no way to judge its adequacy and medical necessity, and often are misled by the . . . fancy gadgets with lights, bells and whistles to suggest safety and state-of-the-art technology;

— lure people into an office by providing something free. The staff believes such ads lead to "hard sell" techniques used once the patient arrives in the office;

— emphasize the reasonableness of fees and the easy financing that's available;

— utilize photographs of attractive models who in most cases have little or no relationship to any cosmetic surgery actually performed by the doctor. The staff believes that psychologically appealing advertising appears to minimize the potential health risks of these surgical procedures; and

— fail to mention even the name of the operating surgeon.

ADVERTISING IN PLASTIC SURGERY
A Position Paper

Congressional Testimony
by Mark Gorney, MD
Past President, American Society of
Plastic and Reconstructive Surgeons

In December 1975, the Federal Trade Commission filed a complaint against the American Medical Association based on the theory that by restricting members from advertising, it was guilty of anti-competitive practices. It was an article of faith of the chief commissioner at the time, Mr. Michael Pertschuk, that advertising would stimulate competition and thus bring down the cost of medical care.

In 1978, the American Society of Plastic and Reconstructive Surgeons was presented with a proposed complaint and consent decree alleging the use of board certification for anti-competitive purposes. We tried by every conceivable means to convince FTC officials that:

A) Such actions would open a Pandora's box—resulting in wholesale, serious injury to the public—since it would strongly encourage those whose greed exceeds their scruples.

B) Removal of controls on physician training and advertising would totally emasculate any disciplinary control medical organizations have over their members.

C) The agency's premise was incorrect, since the forces that shape the marketplace in general do not apply to medicine—regardless of what the "Economics 101" texts say.

D) The FTC was wandering out of its jurisdiction, since we were not arguing about a product but a specialized, highly individualized service that should be denied rather than encouraged for certain individuals . . .

As expected, the last 10 years have brought on a virtual explosion of advertising by all kinds of practitioners who are performing cosmetic surgery. Some advertisers are completely unqualified in plastic surgery, having received their formal training in a field totally unrelated to the specialty. Others have received acceptable training in *certain* plastic surgery procedures, but advertise their willingness to perform operations that fall well outside their documented expertise.

Unfortunately, it is almost impossible for consumers to distinguish between these physicians and fully trained and certified plastic surgeons. Regardless of the fact that they actually received their formal training as an otolaryngologist, dermatologist, gynecologist or other unrelated specialist, these individuals routinely label themselves "plastic surgeons." Those who received certification in their original specialty give themselves a greater veneer of credibility by describing themselves in their ads as "board-certified"—even though their certificate is *not* from the American Board of Plastic Surgery, the *only* body authorized by the American Board of Medical Specialties to certify plastic surgeons.

The average consumer assumes that the federal and state governments are watching out for the public, and that a physician would not be able to call himself a plastic surgeon if he had not completed an extensive program of approved training in that specialty. The average consumer also assumes that if a physician calls himself "board-certified," he has been certified

in the specialty for which he is advertising. Even those sophisticated enough to question this claim, or to look for an ad that
names the specific board, may still be misled when they are
simply told the doctor has been tested by the "American Board
of Cosmetic Surgery." With a name that sounds interchangeable
with the American Board of *Plastic* Surgery, consumers have no
way of knowing that the Cosmetic Board is a different entity,
that it is *not* recognized by the American Board of Medical
Specialties, and that it does *not* require its applicants to complete an accredited residency program in plastic surgery. . . .

This country is filled with unhappy, credulous people "in
search of themselves." On one day, [they] may respond to . . .
astrology, while on the next day they may be vulnerable to a
well-produced advertisement urging that "you owe it to yourself to discover the new you" by getting a new nose, or a larger
pair of breasts. If physicians continue to be allowed to practice
any specialty they wish as long as they have a general medical
degree, then the only way to protect consumers is to give them
the facts they need to make an *informed* choice of practitioner.
. . . We feel strongly that ads designed to persuade uninformed
and credulous laypersons to undergo elective surgical operations that may not even be appropriate for them is not in the
public interest. Many operations in the field of cosmetic plastic
surgery are undoubtedly beneficial both psychologically and
physically for given individuals, while the same operations may
have a disastrous effect on others.

One of the most important functions of surgeons is to
evaluate prospective patients for physical and psychological
suitability and to counsel these impartially. This function is
virtually incompatible with advertising that is primarily designed to "sell" unneeded and unwanted operations before an
initial consultation is held between patient and doctor. Such
advertising, implying that near magical changes in patients'
lives are not only possible but probable, is flourishing in all
states in the union. . . .

As the medical director of the largest malpractice insurance carrier in the West, I can assure you that the computers of the insurance industry are not programmed to distinguish between the trained and the untrained or the scrupulous and the unscrupulous. We fear that if some control is not exerted, the expanding sphere of litigation will adversely affect insurance premiums throughout the specialty.

Anyone who does surgery and claims to never have any complications is a liar, is inexperienced or has a pact with the devil. In the best of hands, complications will occur. However, the one feature that many disastrous results have in common is an absolute lack of discriminatory judgment. Often, the only pre-operative criteria used in these cases were a normal temperature and a valid credit card.

. . . it is harmful to the public to create inflated or unjustified expectations of favorable results; make statements that imply a physician has skills superior to others, unless such skills can be factually substantiated; or use incorrect, incomplete or misleading information that is likely to cause the average person to misunderstand or be deceived. . . . it is the ethical duty of a physician to subordinate financial reward to social responsibility.

. . . the heart of our cases (lies) in a statement made by Chief Justice Burger of the Supreme Court in the Virginia Pharmacy Decision. In language far more eloquent and majestic than we can muster, Justice Burger stated, "I think it important to note . . . that the advertisement of professional services carries with it quite different risks than the advertisement of standard products." Justice Burger then quoted approvingly from an earlier Supreme Court decision prohibiting certain types of advertising by dentists:

"The legislature was not dealing with traders in commodities, but with the vital interests of public health, and with a profession treating bodily ills and demanding different standards of conduct from those which are traditional in the competition of the marketplace. The community is concerned with the maintenance of professional standards which will insure not only competency in individual practitioners, but also protection against those who would prey upon a public peculiarly susceptible to imposition through alluring promises of physical relief. The community is (also) concerned with providing safeguards not only against deception, but against practices which would tend to demoralize the profession by forcing its members into an unseemly rivalry which would enlarge the opportunities of the least scrupulous."

It is evident to us that although it ruled in favor of professional advertising, the Supreme Court of the United States still understood what we feel is at stake. If restrictions and prohibitions on unscrupulous, deceptive advertising are not imposed, the public will respond only to the most costly and excessive displays and end up paying the price. Those physicians who have proven their eagerness to take up the huckster's banner have lost no time in taking advantage of the confusion that exists, thus bringing to life the Supreme Court's vision: "an unseemly rivalry, which would enlarge the opportunities of the least scrupulous."

One hears from FTC officials the opinion that the public benefits of commercial advertising for surgical services outweigh the harm done to a few patients. The American Society of Plastic and Reconstructive Surgeons feels that human life and well-being are precious, and that patients must be protected. It seems to us anomalous to promote a program of advertising that leads to the performance of operations that are inappropriate.

The American Society of Plastic and Reconstructive Surgeons is prepared to document its stand in favor of limits on professional advertising with tragic examples of the human cost of lack of control. These are people who see an ad, respond to it and pay for their innocence the rest of their lives. These are women who ask us with tears in their eyes, "How can this kind of thing be allowed?" The American Society of Plastic and Reconstructive Surgeons asks the same question.

HOSPITAL PEER REVIEW
The Measure of Competence

Congressional Testimony
by Norman M. Cole, MD
Immediate Past President, American Society
of Plastic and Reconstructive Surgeons
Before the House
Subcommittee on Regulation and
Business Opportunities
April 4, 1989

There is a nearly universal public perception that physicians are regulated by state or federal laws which define the training and qualifications of those who present themselves as specialists. If we are to appreciate the current problems which are surfacing in the field of aesthetic (cosmetic) surgery, we must start with a clear understanding that there are no such laws or regulations. . . . The average patient contemplating a surgical procedure is totally unaware of these uncertainties surrounding the very essence of quality care. In virtually every instance where these facts have been presented to the public, the response is predictably incredulous: "How can it be?"

The answer to this question lies in the fact that, until recently, physicians have done a credible job of self-regulation. The moral traditions and ethical standards of the medical profession have engendered a well-deserved trust in the basic edict that a doctor would never lie. . . .

The most meaningful assurance of quality control in plastic surgery is to subject the surgeon's training and experience to the scrutiny of other physicians, both surgeons and non-surgeons. Such scrutiny is called peer review, and it is best accomplished in hospitals by a credentialing process which has been used successfully for many years to assess the competence of every physician or surgeon proposing to practice in the hospital setting.

There is a growing number of physicians whose greed outweighs ethics and concern for patient well-being. They either refuse to accept the decision of their peers or avoid the peer review process altogether, realizing that they do not possess the training or experience to qualify for hospital privileges. Instead, they establish unlicensed and unaccredited surgical facilities in their offices, or build surgical clinics, and aggressively market themselves to an unsuspecting public. The average medical consumer never realizes that these doctors do not meet the standards considered basic and essential by the medical community in order to practice the plastic surgery specialty in an accredited hospital.

An otolaryngologist who operates on a woman to increase the size of her breasts is acting in direct opposition to the American Board of Otolaryngology, which states that such procedures are not within his field of training. He is not performing the procedure from the standpoint of providing a service which is otherwise not available or accommodating the needs of a population which is underserved. He is doing it for the express purpose of personal financial gain . . .

Physicians who perform aesthetic procedures for which they cannot obtain hospital privileges fail, in a very real sense, to meet a community standard. Knowledgeable physicians who are responsible members of hospital credentialing committees recognize the training and qualifications necessary to perform various surgeries, and they will not permit the unqualified to undertake such procedures.

Legislation is urgently needed which will be directed at those who purposely avoid and deny the peer review standards governing the delivery of qualified medical care. These physicians must be required to meet the same standards of training and qualifications that the public expects of hospital-based surgeons. Even if a practitioner intends to perform surgical procedures outside of the hospital setting, the public deserves the assurance that the physician does meet hospital standards and that, if the patient so desired, the physician would be permitted to perform the same procedure in an accredited hospital.

What sort of protection is afforded to the public when a physician who fails to meet hospital standards can remove himself from the hospital setting, set up an unlicensed and unaccredited facility, and represent himself as a specialist in a specialty for which he cannot obtain privileges at a hospital?

The issue is quality care. Peer review is a process which is accepted by every legitimate medical specialty. The day of self-proclaimed specialists must be over, and a new era of concern for public safety must be instituted by meaningful legislation to require every physician claiming to be a specialist to meet hospital standards for that specialty.

THE BREAST IMPLANT CONTROVERSY

INTRODUCTION

In 1976, The Food and Drug Administration was given jurisdiction over medical devices, including breast implants. Sixteen
years later, breast implants were pulled off the market so that
their safety could be evaluated through research.

Sixteen years, with women receiving implants at the average
rate of 100,000 women a year. That's close to 2 million women,
just since 1976. How many women before 1976? No one
knows. Possibly as many as three million women in the United
States have breast implants of one form or another.

Two to three million women are walking around this
country with potential time bombs on their chests.

Or it could be that these millions of women are walking
around with breast implants to which a certain percentage will
prove to be sensitive, to the point of affecting their health. Or,
the normal bodily reactions of some, maybe only a few, of
these women will cause their systems to overreact. Let's say
some of these women have a genetic propensity for diseases
such as scleroderma or arthritis—maybe they will prematurely
begin to suffer from these diseases. Or maybe the ubiquitous

presence of a foreign substance in the form of silicone gel actually *causes* these diseases, or creates a situation in the body in which there's so much silicone to get rid of that the body becomes allergic to itself.

Then again research may prove silicone to be harmless.

Anecdotal evidence appears to support that many women are uncomfortably sensitive to their breast implants.

Capsular contracture, or the hardening of the breasts, is simply a normal bodily response to the introduction of a foreign body. Just as an oyster will form a pearl from a piece of sand, the human body will wall off a foreign body to prevent it from polluting the rest of the system. The degree of hardness in a breast implant and its resultant physical or aesthetic discomfort can only be assessed by the taste of the wearer. Hardness for some is welcome firmness for others.

Autoimmune diseases, however, are life-threatening and debilitating. To date, research shows only a *possible* link between breast implants and autoimmune or connective tissue diseases. It is not known whether sufferers were prone to these diseases anyway. It has been shown, however, that the condition of scleroderma sufferers improves remarkably when the implants are removed.

Implants coated with polyurethane, a substance which even the manufacturer warned shouldn't be used in the human body, is broken down almost immediately after it is introduced into the body, producing a chemical called TDA. Products such as hair dyes containing TDA had already been pulled off the market because of the chemical's known carcinogenicity and its suspected link with birth defects. TDA has been found not only in the urine, but also the breast milk of women with these implants, raising the specter of adverse effects on future generations.

Silicone has been used in biomedical products for many years. Considered to be biologically inert by many scientists, silicone's usefulness has advanced medical technology and helped countless people who have needed artificial parts for their hearts, dialysis, prostheses for their fingers, toes, and limbs. But is it really inert? Our government recently decreed that asbestos be removed from buildings, schools, and private homes because of its link to cancer. The average time for cancer to appear after exposure to asbestos is 37 years. In comparison, the effects of silicone have been studied for a maximum period of 10 to 12 years. It's possible that this biologically inert substance simply has a long latency period for causing cancer. We have no way of knowing—yet.

With technological advances come high-tech problems.

What took the FDA so long to insist that implants be tested for safety? For one thing, other products took precedence. For another, breast implants had been used for about fifteen years prior to coming under the FDA's jurisdiction, with few reported problems. The medical lobby, a very strong influence, allegedly played a role. Even now, doctors scoff at the possible dangers of breast implants.

Another mystifying fact is that the FDA has placed a moratorium on silicone gel breast implants, but not silicone gel calf implants nor pectoral implants for men which are constructed identically to those placed in women's bodies. Could this really be a paternalistic issue?

As to the toxicity of silicone in the body, Dr. Larry Seifert says, "It ought to be appreciated that one of the central elements in it is silicon, the second most plentiful element on the planet Earth and the second or third most plentiful in the universe; a trace element in all of our bodies and in the foods we eat and in the L.A. water supply, and that silicone is prevalent in an industrial society. It's in hairspray, it's in the lipstick you're wearing right now. Bite or lick your lips, swallow it nervously, it goes in your stomach, it's absorbed by the cells. It's in pacemakers, it's in heart valves, it's in newsprint, it's in a variety of antacids where it's called simethicone."

But in none of these products can you find the comparatively enormous amount of loose silicone that would be released from a leaking or ruptured breast implant. How many antacid tablets would you have to consume to put an equivalent amount of silicone in your body? Could it be possible that the toxicity of silicone is directly proportional to the amount ingested by the cells?

In terms of having implants removed, all sides discourage the explantation of a non-problematic implant. All sides recommend that a ruptured or leaking implant be removed. Many doctors say that breasts will look deformed if implants are not replaced. Other doctors say that the breasts will simply look the same as they did before the implants were inserted. Some of the doctors are saying the same thing in two different ways.

Doctors claim that the FDA doesn't really believe that silicone gel implants cause either cancer or diseases related to the immune system. They may be right. Considering the FDA's decision to pull silicone gel breast implants off the market pending further study, we see that gel implants are still allowed for reconstruction patients. "Reconstruction" is a term applied to procedures which create normalcy for someone who suffers from an abnormality due to a birth or developmental defect, or from the loss of a breast from cancer or other accident.

How can the FDA allow women who have already suffered the devastating loss of a breast from cancer to further risk their lives and health with a product that has never been properly tested for safety, and which may yet be found to cause cancer itself? The ruling makes absolutely no sense.

Looking a little deeper, women suffering from "micromastia" can conceivably still go to their doctors for treatment of this congenital or developmental deformity and receive treatment in the form of silicone gel breast implants, since the correction of a deformity would be considered "reconstruction."

I wonder how small-breasted a woman has to be to qualify for treatment of micromastia. Considering the American fascination with large breasts, perhaps a B-cup?

Why would anyone want to have their breasts augmented anyway? Who benefits? Certainly not a nursing child. This book is not about gender issues, but perhaps an assessment of priorities versus fashion could be made when the lives of three million American women may be at stake.

On the other hand, statistics show that most women with breast implants are very happy and would have it done again without a second thought. Except bigger.

Women must be allowed power over their own bodies. But should they also be allowed the use of an improperly tested, potentially unhealthy product? Should autonomy also extend to drugs; are laws against crack cocaine to be considered "paternalistic" because of the tragic proliferation of crack babies?

Women will be able to make intelligent choices only when all of the research information about breast implants is accessible to them. Paternalism enters the issue when that information is interpreted variously by interest groups, particularly those who stand to make money from breast implants.

STAMPING OUT A DREAD SCOURGE

by Barbara Ehrenreich

Time Magazine
February 17, 1992

In the spirit of a public health campaign, the American Society of Plastic and Reconstructive Surgeons (ASPRS) has launched a p.r. drive to "tell the other side of the [breast implant] story." Public health? Slicing women's chests open so that they can be stuffed with a close chemical relative of Silly Putty? Yes, indeed, because the plastic surgeons understand what the FDA is so reluctant to acknowledge: small breasts are not just a harmless challenge to the bikini wearer or would-be topless entertainer. They are a disease, a disfiguring illness for which the technical term is micromastia.

As the ASPRS tried to explain to the FDA almost 10 years ago, "There is a substantial and enlarging body of medical information and opinion to the effect that these deformities [small breasts] are really a disease." Not a fatal disease, perhaps, to judge from the number of sufferers who are still hobbling around untreated, but a disease nonetheless, like the flu or TB. And anyone tempted to fault the establishment for inaction on breast cancer or AIDS should consider its quiet but no less heroic progress against the scourge of micromastia: in the past

30 years, 1.6 million victims have been identified and cured. Who says our health system doesn't work?

Once we understand that small breasts are a "disease," it's easier to see why Dow Corning and others rushed so breathlessly to get their implants onto the market. Why diddle around with slow, costly tests while an epidemic is raging out there? And everyone's life is touched by the tragedy of micromastia because everyone has a friend, sister, co-worker or wife who falls pitifully short in the mammary department. In the past, small groups of health-conscious males, typically gathered at construction sites, would offer free diagnoses to women passersby, but there was little that could be done until the advent of the insertable Silly Putty breast.

Admittedly, micromastia is in some ways an atypical disease. It is painless, which is why many victims put off treatment for years, and it in no way diminishes breast function, if that is still defined as lactation. The implants, on the other hand, can interfere with lactation, and they make mammograms less able to find cancer (not to mention the potential for a disfiguring or life-threatening side effect like lupus or scleroderma). But so what if micromastia has no functional impact? Why can't a disease be manifested solely by size?

. . . Though nearly 2 million micromastia victims have been cured, millions more remain untreated, as shown by the continued existence of the plague's dread symbol - the A-cup bra. There have been many earnest attempts to reach the untreated: public health-oriented magazines like *Playboy,* for example, repeatedly print photos illustrating normal breast size for the woman in doubt. Tragically, though, many women still live in denial, concealing their condition under mannish blazers and suit jackets, forgoing the many topless forms of employment.

Now a cynic might see the silicone-implant business as another malfeasance on the scale of the Dalkon Shield (which had a tendency to cause devastating infections) [or] DES (which could cause cancer in the user's offspring) . . . A cynic might point to the medical profession's long habit of exploiting the female body for profit - from the 19th century custom of removing the ovaries as a cure for "hysteria" to our more recent traditions of unnecessary hysterectomies and caesarians. A cynic might conclude that the real purpose of the $500 million-a-year implant business is the implantation of fat in the bellies and rumps of underemployed plastic surgeons.

But our cynic would be missing the point of modern medical science. We may not have a cure for every disease, alas, but there's no reason we can't have a disease for every cure. With silicone implants, small breasts become micromastia. . . . Plastic surgeons can now cure sagging jowls and chins, droopy eyelids and insufficiently imposing male chests and calves. So we can expect to hear soon about the menace of new diseases such as saggy-jowlitis and hypopectoralis.

It will be hard, though, to come up with anything quite so convincing as micromastia. As the plastic surgeons must have realized, American culture is almost uniquely obsessed with large, nurturing bosoms. And with the silicone scandal upon us, we can begin to see why: in a society so unnurturing that even health care can sadistically be perverted for profit, people are bound to have a desperate, almost pathological need for the breast.

FROM PUBLIC CITIZEN HEALTH RESEARCH GROUP

Memo from Sidney Wolfe, MD

From: Public Citizen, November 9, 1988
To: Frank Young, MD., Ph.D., Commissioner, FDA

We have obtained internal Dow Corning and FDA documents that contain information already well known to you, which clearly demonstrate that silicone gel, currently being implanted in 130,000 women a year in the form of breast implants, causes highly malignant cancers in over 23% of the animals tested. According to one of the FDA memos, "while there is no direct proof that silicone causes cancers in humans, there is considerable reason to suspect that it can do so." As you well know, animal evidence of carcinogenicity is regarded as posing a risk of cancer in humans. In light of this evidence, I urge you to halt immediately the use of silicone gel materials for implantation into the human body. . . .

FDA should also promptly investigate why the detailed records of the Dow Corning study . . . which show silicone gel to be carcinogenic were apparently not promptly sent to FDA but were obtained during an FDA inspection of DOW in December, 1987.

You must explain why six and one-half years elapsed before finalizing the FDA's January 19, 1982 proposal to require Dow and other companies making silicone gel breast implants to submit safety data on this product because, as stated in 1982, it *"presents a potential unreasonable risk of injury."*. . .

Sincerely,

Sidney M. Wolfe, M.D.,
Director, Public Citizen Health Research Group

Reprinted by kind permission of Public Citizen Health Research Group. Their publication, *Health Letter,* can be obtained for $18 per year by writing to Public Citizen, 2000 P Street NW, Washington, DC 20036.

Animal Testing and Cancer
by Sidney Wolfe, MD

Testimony of Sidney M. Wolfe, MD

Director, Public Citizen Health Research Group

Washington D.C.

before FDA Advisory Committee

on General and Plastic Surgery Devices

. . . Animals are the only way we have of predicting and preventing human cancer. Animal studies can only predict whether or not cancer will occur in humans, not, very accurately, the magnitude of the risk. The tragic story of animal studies, in 1938, showing that DES, later to be widely used to prevent miscarriages, caused cancer should not have to be repeated. Because doctors and the drug companies did not pay attention to animal evidence, thousands of women got vaginal or cervical cancer (DES daughters) or breast cancer (DES mothers).

. . .

In an internal FDA review . . . FDA staffers concluded that "silicone can migrate to other body sites away from the site of implantation. Even with all the biases inherent in the study design, the authors did note a higher number of observed cases of cancers at other sites than expected (24 observed versus 15.8 expected). Based on these results and the fact that silicone can migrate to other sites, the authors should have addressed this issue by including cancers at other sites, instead of limiting their study to only breast cancer."

When I asked National Cancer Institute epidemiologist Robert Hoover, M.D., who had been a member of the NIH/FDA ad hoc committee whether the extension of the follow-up to

10-12 years ruled out the possibility of human cancer as Dr. Brody and others would have us believe, he replied that all it shows is that at an average follow-up (for all of the women) of this long, no breast cancer has showed up. That this does not offer much solace, based on what is known about human cancer, is seen in the following table:

Average Number of Years After Exposure Before Human Cancer Occurs*

Carcinogen	Type of Cancer	Avg Latency
Chromium	Lung Cancer	20-25 years
Radium	Bone Sarcoma	23 yrs (high dose)
Radium	Bone Sarcoma	35 yrs (low dose)
Vinyl Chloride	Liver Angiosarcoma	21 years
Nickel	Lung Cancer	24 years
Aromatic Amines	Bladder Cancer	14-45 years
Hardwood Dusts	Nasal Cancer	30 years
Asbestos	Mesothelioma	37 years
Silicone Gel Breast Implants	The average # of Years of Follow up	**10-12 years**

. . .

In addition to the paper in the *JAMA*, July 8, 1988 . . . another study on connective tissue disease associated with the use of silicone gel breast implants was recently reported at the Western meeting of the American Rheumatology Association by three rheumatologists from UCLA, Weiner, Clements and Paulus. They had previously reported 3 cases of chronic arthritis after silicone gel implants . . . In the more recent study, they reported 8 more cases and stated that "these 11 cases suggest a possible relationship between silicone gel implants and the later development of connective tissue disease."

*Public Citizen Health Research Group adapted from Dr. Richard Hayes 13th International Cancer Conference 1982.

Silicone Breast Implants Are Associated With Immune Diseases
by Douglas Teich, MD

Statement by Dr. Douglas Teich

Hearing before FDA's General and Plastic

Surgical Devices Committee, January 26, 1989

There have now been some 69 reported cases of connective tissue disease, chronic arthritis or auto-immune disorder following cosmetic surgery involving injection or implantation of silicone or other foreign material. Twelve cases have been described in patients receiving paraffin injections, 31 in patients injected with silicone, silicone and paraffin, or uncertain mixtures, and 26 patients had received silicone gel or saline-filled silicone elastomeric envelope-type implants.

21 cases of scleroderma (or its variants, such as morphea) have been published, of which 10 come from Japan or Singapore. We have a pre-print abstract from rheumatologists in Southern California reporting that, now that a possible association is more widely appreciated, they have located some 23 additional patients with scleroderma or its variants having had augmentation mammoplasty simply by mailing and reviewing a questionnaire sent to members of the United Scleroderma Foundation.

. . . The latency period has ranged from two months to 25 years, with most cases occurring 10 to 15 years after the procedure. These women are not usually seen for such prob-

Courtesy of *Public Citizen*.

lems by the plastic surgeon who performed the procedure; rather, they seek the attention of their primary care physician or internist, or are referred to a dermatologist or rheumatologist, and, often, the fact that cosmetic surgery was performed years before is overlooked.

. . . there have been several documented instances of remission following the removal of what may be the offending immunologic stimulus. The remissions occurring in those patients with scleroderma are particularly striking, since spontaneous sustained improvements are most unusual in patients with advanced disease of the native variety.

. . . Complete and lengthy follow-up is . . . critical in studies of diseases with long latency periods. . . . There is enough evidence that significant immune derangement, with consequent connective tissue disease, occurs with exposure to the silicone in breast implants to warrant careful epidemiologic study. Until either a well-designed case control study or a cohort study with enough patients and lengthy follow-up proves otherwise, these implants are not safe for human use.

HOW INDUSTRIAL FOAM CAME TO BE EMPLOYED IN BREAST IMPLANTS

By Thomas M. Burton

Staff Reporter of *The Wall Street Journal*

March 25, 1992

Harold Markham built a successful family business selling what appeared to be a better breast implant.

Mr. Markham's implant, like most others used in the past two decades, was essentially a bag of silicone gel. Ordinary silicone-gel implants, doctors knew, in some cases could slip out of position or cause breast tissue to harden. But the Markham Implant was covered in a layer of spongy polyurethane foam, which tended to prevent these problems.

The Markham implant worked so well that by the late 1980s it became an industry leader; an estimated 200,000 were sold in the U.S. alone. The business was acquired in 1988 by Bristol-Myers Squibb Co., and Mr. Markham retired in Beverly Hills, Calif., flush with the success of his polyurethane lining, described in company documents as the "patented Microthane interface system."

The lining actually has another name: Scott Industrial Foam. It is used in automobile air filters and carpet-cleaning equipment. In the human body, tests have found it can degrade into a substance called 2,4-toluene diamine, or TDA, a chemical that is suspected of causing cancer in humans. The foam's manufacturer, Scotfoam Corp. of Eddystone, Pa., says that it was never intended for use in medical applications.

When Scotfoam officials discovered in 1987 that it was being surgically implanted in women, they told the implant manufacturer that Scotfoam didn't recommend its product to be used in people. But the foam continued to be implanted—until last year, when the Food and Drug Administration for the first time asked breast-implant makers to submit data showing their products were safe.

It isn't known whether TDA is released into the body by the polyurethane-coated implants in sufficient quantity to cause cancer. Bristol-Myers maintains that the implants are "safe and effective," but after the FDA issued its request for safety data the company withdrew the implants from the market, saying that further, time-consuming research would be needed to prove their safety. As a result, Bristol-Myers avoided the intense scrutiny that other makers of silicone-gel implants received during the recent FDA breast-implant hearings. Bristol-Myers says it is currently conducting tests to determine the effects of polyurethane in the body.

Women who received the Markham implants—marketed under such brand names as Meme, Natural Y and Replicon—face the same health questions that have been raised about the silicone gel in ordinary implants, including suspected links to autoimmune-system disorders. The problem of polyurethane degradation adds another set of concerns. TDA is classified by the U.S. government as a hazardous waste, and it was banned for use in hair dyes in 1971. Workers who handle it are advised to wear goggles, rubber gloves and respirators. TDA has been found in both the breast milk and the urine of women with polyurethane-coated implants.

Mr. Markham, now 73 years old, declines to be interviewed. He has said repeatedly that his products are safe.

With little oversight by federal regulators, energetic salesmen like Mr. Markham had an open field in the 1970s and the

1980s to sell medical implants. Medical devices were essentially unregulated by the FDA until 1976, and scrutiny of them was minimal for years afterward. An FDA official expressed concern about the Markham implant in 1981, and warned that some polyurethanes might be carcinogenic, but the agency didn't take action.

Mr. Markham, like many executives of medical-supply companies, has no formal medical training. Born in New York City and known to friends as Hal, he served in the Army medical corps after World War II and for a time sold chewing gum for Wm. Wrigley Jr. Co. He was working as a medical-supply salesman in 1970 when he met John Pangman, the Beverly Hills surgeon who invented the foam-covered implant.

Dr. Pangman is dead, and it isn't clear just what led him to try covering a silicone-gel implant with foam.   Franklin L. Ashley, an early researcher on the foam-covered implant, explained in medical-journal articles in 1970 and 1972 that it held its shape and maintained its position in the breast better. But another, unforeseen advantage became apparent in time.

Other breast implants then on the market had a smooth silicone lining around the goopy silicone gel. Some women's bodies reacted to the silicone lining by forming a kind of human-tissue capsule around it, as if to wall off the foreign invader. This "capsular contracture" led to misshapen breasts and painful hardening in 5% to 10% of women who received ordinary implants; the rate was cut to 2% to 3% by the foam lining, according to Scott L. Spear, professor of plastic surgery at Georgetown University Medical Center in Washington, D.C. Evidently, contracture was reduced because the foam had lots of holes for human tissue to grow into.

In time, the downside of this feature would become apparent, too: If the implant ruptured—and some did—removing it "could be a bear," as one Markham salesman testified in a 1991 New York liability lawsuit.

Mr. Markham seized upon Dr. Pangman's idea and arranged to have the implant produced in volume by Heyer-Schulte

Corp., a medical-device concern based in Santa Barbara, Calif. He set up a tiny sales staff, including his wife and daughter, to begin marketing the new devices.

Eventually, however, Heyer-Schulte officials lost faith in both Mr. Markham and his implant. Thomas Talcott, then director of materials research at Heyer-Schulte and now a prominent critic of the breast-implant industry, says the implant sometimes caused a "gross inflammatory response." (Robert S. Niemann, an attorney for Mr. Markham, says any such responses were short-term.)

James Rudy, then president of Heyer-Schulte, says he, too, was concerned by reports of inflammation. "I felt I was in the process of lending my company's name to a device I couldn't defend," he says. And, he says, "I felt Markham claimed personal expertise that he didn't have." He acknowledges that no one at Heyer-Schulte ever checked the foam's chemical makeup.

In the mid-1970s, Heyer-Schulte officials grew concerned enough about the polyurethane implant that they decided to stop making it. Mr. Markham in 1978 persuaded Mr. Rudy to turn over the Pangman patent to him, for free.

Alistair Winn, another former Heyer-Schulte aide, says Mr. Markham increasingly grew devoted to the virtues of the polyurethane product. "The first thing that comes to mind about Hal Markham is mind over matter—he strongly believes in his product," says Mr. Winn. "When doctors would ask him about the breakdown of the polyurethane, he would say it doesn't matter and that it works fine in people," Mr. Winn says. "He didn't know he was right. He would just tell the world what it wanted to hear."

Mr. Markham has repeatedly maintained his products are safe. He cites a oxicologist Marc Lappe concluded that TDA caused a benign tumor to become malignant and grow more rapidly in a New York computer programmer who sued the makers of the po yurethane implant. Dr. Lappe, a consultant t concluded that none had shown any signs of cancer.

But Dr. Brand also said the polyurethane cover didn't break

down in the mice, a phenomenon that surgeons say they *have* frequently seen in women. A 1982 report by Walter Reed Army Medical Center researchers in Washington, for instance, found that in one patient "there was nearly complete disintegration and absorption of the polyurethane foam cover" over a nine-year period. Dr. Brand acknowledges today that "my observation time [was] too short. We do not have controlled studies on the polyurethane over time." He says it isn't known whether his mice would have been exposed to TDA had the study lasted longer.

There isn't any evidence that Mr. Markham did anything beyond Dr. Brand's study to learn the chemical makeup of the product. His daughter, Jacqueline, who has a master's degree in fine arts from UCLA, was his company's "vice president of technical and scientific affairs and applications" and later its president. But when she was asked in a 1988 deposition whether she or her father knew the composition of the material in the implants, she answered, "Gosh, no." Jacqueline Markham declined to be interviewed; the deposition was part of a civil case in New York federal court brought against one of Mr. Markham's companies, Natural Y Surgical Specialties Inc., by a woman who contended she had contracted cancer from the implants. A jury awarded her $4.45 million in damages; a judge set aside part of that award, and the two sides subsequently settled for more than $1 million.

Mr. Markham marketed the implant through Natural Y, based in Los Angeles. With an initial capitalization of $80,000, he also became a co-owner of Aesthetech Corp., a company based in Paso Robles, Calif., that was set up to manufacture the implant.

Mr. Markham's sales force spurred business through marketing pitches that were clever, aggressive, and sometimes misleading. "Reasonable care was used in the choice of materials and manufacture of this product," said one sales brochure supplied to plastic surgeons. Salesmen told surgeons the foam was cut with lasers, an assertion that has been contradicted in court testimony.

Also helpful in boosting sales was an article by New York plastic surgeon Steven Herman in the journal *Plastic and Reconstructive Surgery*. He wrote: "The Meme implant has been found to be eminently satisfactory. Its disadvantage is that it is more easily ruptured during placement, but it produces a breast that is esthetically pleasing and, in every instance thus far, a breast that is free of firmness and capsular contracture."

He didn't mention his own relationship to Mr. Markham's Natural Y. Mr. Markham later testified, in a 1988 case filed against Aesthetech in Harris County, Texas, district court, that Dr. Herman received 3.5% of the revenue from sales of the Meme implant. Dr. Herman didn't respond to repeated requests for comment. (He is not to be confused with Stephen Herman, also a New York doctor, who is a psychiatrist.)

Scotfoam officials say they first learned that their product was being used in breast implants because of a Florida liability lawsuit over the device. As part of the discovery process in that case, University of Florida chemist Christopher Batich broke down the foam chemically and found that TDA, a known animal carcinogen and a suspected human one, was produced. (While the hydrolysis experiment was done at high temperature, other, more recent studies designed to more closely mimic body processes also found TDA.)

On Dec. 2, 1987, Thomas Powell, a co-owner of Aesthetech, called Scotfoam to ask whether this was possible. Scotfoam product control manager Edward Griffiths told him that it was. "We were shocked" to learn the foam was being used in implants, Mr. Griffiths says. Two days later, Mr. Griffiths wrote himself a memo about the call: "I explained our position on implants," Mr. Griffiths wrote. "Namely, we do not recommend such uses."

Scotfoam also informed Aesthetech that TDA is routinely produced as a by-product in the foaming reaction that makes the polyurethane. Tests done for Scotfoam—which is affiliated with a private company called 21 International Holdings Inc.—

have detected TDA in the final foam product, though the company says the testing procedures might have contributed to TDA formation.

But Aesthetech continued to use Scott Industrial Foam, and sales of the Markham implant continued to soar. Aesthetech was bought by Cooper Cos., a New York health-care conglomerate, in 1987; in December 1988 Cooper sold Aesthetech to Bristol-Myers's Surgitek unit. Bristol-Myers declined to comment on whether it had been informed of any health-related questions about the foam when it made the acquisition.

The first sign of any concern about the Markham implants at the FDA had occurred back in 1981. On Oct. 26 of that year, Thomas V. Kelley, a consumer safety officer for the FDA, wrote to the agency's investigations branch in Los Angeles suggesting that it pay a visit to Markham's Natural Y Surgical Specialties office in Los Angeles and determine the foam's chemical content. Mr. Kelley said in his memorandum that the agency "has reason to believe that the prosthesis is covered with a polyurethane foam which may tend to disintegrate. . . . In addition, certain polyurethanes are known to be carcinogenic."

FDA investigators did visit Mr. Markham, at least three times in the following years. But the agency didn't follow through on Mr. Kelley's original suspicion. Instead, the visits concerned routine requests for administrative information. Agency officials didn't learn anything more about the chemical content of the foam until Prof. Batich wrote to them about finding TDA as a byproduct of its degradation.

The FDA itself within the past two years conducted a test to see what the polyurethane disintegrates into, and found that TDA was indeed produced. Alan Andersen, science director in the FDA's medical devices center, says the agency's early indications are that there is a "relatively low risk" of cancer produced by the polyurethane, but adds, "We believe this is real."

Bristol-Myers says it believes that the TDA found in the tests may somehow have been artificially created through the testing methodologies. The company has criticized one common TDA testing method, called acid hydrolysis, because it employs acid and intense (150-degree Centigrade) heat. But even recent tests using methods designed for Bristol-Myers also found that the foam degraded into TDA.

In one, Nashville forensic toxicologist David L. Black, using an organic solvent, found TDA in the breast milk of a woman with foam implants. Bristol-Myers criticizes this test, too, as using acid and heat; Dr. Black's method uses 70-degree Centigrade heat, not on the milk itself but at the tail end of the analysis. "Bristol-Myers felt this procedure was entirely reliable until we happened to find toluene diamine in some breast milk," says Dr. Black, who did earlier TDA research for Bristol-Myers. The firm now has proposed to the FDA a new test method for future research.

Scores of lawsuits, naming various defendants, have been filed by women alleging they got cancer or other maladies as a result of the polyurethane-coated implants.

Recently, TDA has been detected in the urine of patients with polyurethane implants. Michael Szycher, a Boston engineer who has testified as an expert witness for implant makers, performed tests for Bristol-Myers and also found TDA formed when the foam broke down in ways designed to mimic body processes. But he concluded the amount was "insignificant" and deems the product safe.

In contrast, University of Illinois at Chicago pathologist and toxicologist Marc Lappe concluded that TDA caused a benign tumor to become malignant and grow more rapidly in a New York computer programmer who sued the makers of the polyurethane implant. Dr. Lappe, a consultant to the FDA's advisory panel on medical devices—and an expert witness for plaintiffs in breast-implant lawsuits—testified at the 1991 trial of her case in New York federal court that polyurethane foam implants are "unfit and unsafe, until proven otherwise, for implantation in the human body."

EVIDENCE FOR THE CARCINOGENICITY OF SILICONE GEL IMPLANTS

Dr. Sidney M. Wolfe, Editor

Health Letter
December 1988, Vol. 4, No.12

The two-year rat carcinogenicity study which was done by Dow Corning to see if silicone gel caused cancer involved three groups of animals, each with 50 males and 50 females. The first group (the controls) developed no malignant fibrosarcoma tumors similar to the ones seen in the silicone-treated animals. One of the other two groups was implanted with a silicone gel used before 1976 and 20 percent of the females and 22 percent of the males developed fibrosarcomas at the injection site. Even more worrisome, 21 percent of the animals with these tumors had evidence that the cancer had spread, including to lungs, kidney, adrenal glands, skin, thymus, and liver. The third group was implanted with the silicone gel currently in use and in this group, 23 percent of the females and 26 percent of the males had gel-associated fibrosarcomas. In 18 percent of the animals, sarcomas spread to distant organs including the heart, lung, liver, pancreas, stomach, and thymus. It was also found that in 85 percent of all of the animals with fibrosarcomas, the tumor caused the death of the animal.

. . . Robert Sheridan, Acting Director of the Office of Device

Reprinted by kind permission of The Public Citizen Health Research Group.

Evaluation [at Dow], stated that: "Dow Corning agrees that silicone gel is sarcomagenic [can cause tumors]. However, this sponsor contends that induction of sarcoma in rats is due to solid-state [caused by a foreign object] carcinogenesis. . . . This is uniquely a rodent phenomenon. Therefore . . . it is of no human health consequence as solid-state cancer in man has not been documented. . . .

FDA staffers, on the other hand, noted the following:

- Solid-state tumor has been reported in rats, mice, chickens, rabbits, and dogs. *It is biologically unconvincing that man is a uniquely resistant species.*

- The cited [by Dow] epidemiological study is severely flawed. The major deficiency of the study is that mean follow-up time is about five years which is nowhere near the two-thirds of life-time required for tumor induction in rats.

- The sarcomas [tumors] in the rat study are at variance with several classical characteristics of solid-state tumor. They are highly metastatic [likely to spread], lethal and show no variation between sexes.

- The event of induction of sarcoma in 25% of test animals is a very important observation as it is lethal in 85% of the sarcomatous animals. This should be viewed in the context that sufficient time has not elapsed to record epidemiologically significant increase in human malignancies. . . . even though the silicone gel is encased in a silicone envelope when used in breast prostheses, . . . silicone gel "bleeds" through the envelope and can thus get to other places in the body. "Silicone gel-filled breast implants allow slow diffusion of gel through the silicone elastomer shell into surrounding tissues. . . . Many investigators have reported on the finding of silicone in lymph nodes and an associated lymphadenopathy [inflammation of the lymph nodes] in women who had undergone mammoplasty [breast augmentation or reconstruction] with silicone, either by injection or by placement of gel-filled prostheses."

SILICONE BREAST IMPLANTS ARE ASSOCIATED WITH IMMUNE DISEASES

from Public Citizen Health Letter

Silicone gel, implanted in 130,000 American women a year in the form of breast implants, has been shown to cause a highly malignant form of cancer in laboratory animals.

. . . another possible long-term health hazard must be added to the all-too-common local complications of these implants. There have been many recent reports of a wide range of "autoimmune diseases," in which the body's immune system is affected (perhaps "boosted") by the presence of silicone gel, which has leaked out of the implant itself, into the surrounding tissues and draining lymph glands, sometimes migrating to distant parts of the body. It appears that the free silicone (or other substances associated with its manufacture) may cause the body to recognize its own parts as "foreign," and mount an attack on its own joints, skin, mucous membranes and other connective tissues (body support structures). This attack can take the form of scleroderma, with thickened, hard skin of the face and hands, eventually involving the entire body and internal organs, or chronic arthritis, with stiff, aching joints which may become swollen and deformed.

Although the original reports of these and related conditions were in Japanese women who had received injections of silicone, paraffin, and other substances, the same types of disease have now been reported in American women several months to 25 years after receiving silicone gel or saline-filled, silicone rubber-type envelope implants.

. . .

The Dow Corning Corporation, the major manufacturer of silicone gel, has amassed *30 years'* worth of research on the biosafety of implanted materials, including silicone and silicone gel. At an FDA hearing on January 26, 1989, a company representative stated that Dow Corning had submitted information to the FDA that included, among other items, "a summary list of 750 biosafety studies conducted by or on behalf of Dow Corning; pooled reports on 39 toxicology studies; and a final report on the two-year Industrial Biotest Labs study conducted from 1976 to 1978 [a highly disputed study which demonstrated that silicone gel produced malignant tumors of the lymphatic system]."

On January 27[1] the Public Citizen Health Research Group requested access to all of the information comprising Dow Corning's biosafety research, under the Freedom of Information Act. When the FDA did not respond within the 10 working days allowed, on February 14 the Public Citizen Litigation Group brought suit against the agency in the United States District Court for the District of Columbia and, subsequently, filed a motion for a temporary restraining order to prevent the FDA from returning some of these documents to Dow.

. . .

It is tragic that we must sue our government to obtain information about the safety of a device that has been implanted in more than two million women in this country. This is information that the FDA should have required (and that should have been subject to outside review), as part of a pre-market approval process, some 25 years ago.[2]

---

[1] 1988.

[2] Editor's note: The FDA only acquired jurisdiction over medical devices, including breast implants, in 1976. Therefore, the FDA could not have required pre-market approval of any medical device in use prior to that time—KO

CONFLICT AND ACTION
CONGRESS vs FDA

One Hundred Second Congress
Congress of the United States
House of Representatives
Human Resources and Intergovernmental
Relations Subcommittee of the Committee on
Government Operations

Rayburn House Office Building, Room B-372
Washington, DC 20515

April 26, 1991

David A. Kessler, M.D.
Commissioner
Food and Drug Administration
Rockville, MD 20857

Dear Dr. Kessler:

. . . As I mentioned on Tuesday, the subcommittee has had difficulty obtaining documents it has requested regarding these implants for almost one year. FDA responses to our requests have improved recently, but we again had problems with our last request, which pertained specifically to polyurethane covered implants.

The documents received on Wednesday, several of which

will be made part of the hearing record, reveal that the most recent public FDA statements on these implants *do not accurately reflect the conclusions of FDA's own scientists*. In fact, *the cancer risks* of TDA released by the polyurethane *may be more than 100 times* the levels reported by FDA and by Surgitek, the manufacturer.

Equally worrisome, the FDA's recent public announcements did not even mention the *risks of birth defects* that were associated with TDA in animals in 1975. These risks were well known to FDA, since they contributed to removing hair dyes with TDA in the 1970's. They are especially important because most women with implants are of childbearing age, and they have been told it is safe to nurse their infants.

These inconsistencies, between the actions of FDA officials and the concerns of FDA's own scientists, are unfortunately similar to the pattern that I discussed with FDA's witnesses at our Congressional hearing in December. FDA's documents indicate that for more than ten years, FDA scientists expressed concerns about the safety of silicone breast implants that were *frequently ignored by FDA officials*. In addition, very serious scientific concerns about the polyurethane implants were obvious in FDA internal documents for several years. Nevertheless, silicone breast implants were not categorized as Class III medical devices until 1988, and the final rule requiring manufacturers to provide safety data was not published until April 10 of this year. Even then, the polyurethane covered implant was not treated differently than the other silicone gel implants, although safety data regarding TDA was mentioned in the final rule.

An FDA memorandum, dated April 2, 1981, indicates that a study conducted by Surgitek several years ago, which the company had failed to make available to FDA in a timely manner, indicates that polyurethane implanted in rats had disintegrated by 50% within six months. Since the amount of the carcinogen TDA released by the breast implant is associated with the disintegration of the polyurethane, these results mean that the levels of TDA would be greater in the human body than in the lab study conducted by FDA.

When the media reported some of the concerns raised at the April 11 meeting, I fear that some at FDA became more concerned about the reputation of the manufacturer than informing the public. While I agree with FDA statements reassuring women with polyurethane implants that they should not panic, I strongly disagree with FDA's public statements that misrepresented the concerns of FDA scientists. American women deserve better.

- FDA did not mention that TDA caused genetic defects in animals. In fact, hair dyes containing TDA were removed from the market in the 1970's due to concerns about the potential for cancer, birth defects and miscarriages. Information about these dangers should be made available immediately to women with implants who may be pregnant or nursing infants.

- FDA officials emphasized the fact that TDA is proven to cause cancer in animals, but not in humans. They neglected to mention that the same is true for most carcinogens that are banned or regulated in the U.S. In fact, TDA is listed as a positive animal carcinogen and potential (or anticipated) human carcinogen by FDA, EPA, and OSHA, as well as the National Toxicology Program and the International Agency for Research on Cancer (IARC).

- FDA emphasized that the amount of TDA found in their studies was very small, a relative term. The amounts are small, but the FDA study indicated that the amounts increase steadily over time. They were studied for approximately one month; the results suggest that the amount would greatly increase over a period of years. In addition, infection or other changes in body conditions could increase the amount of TDA released. Surgitek's own rat study (mentioned above) shows that the level of TDA is likely to increase greatly over time.

- The FDA officials also said that their study found that the polyurethane "might degrade" into TDA. In fact, the FDA scientists concluded that it does degrade into TDA.

- The FDA press release suggested that concerned patients and doctors should call Surgitek for information. This is the classic case of the fox giving advice to the chickens on how to protect themselves. For example, Surgitek claims that they know of not one single case of cancer from their product, although a jury recently awarded $4.4 million to a woman who was adjudged to have cancer due to her Surgitek implant.

- It is also worth noting that, according to agency staff, Surgitek's own study was terminated prematurely when the results appeared damaging, and that the company may be guilty of improper conduct in refusing to provide the final report to FDA.

During the last 25 years, more than two million American women have been subjected to virtually unregulated use of different types of silicone breast implants.

I am writing to urge you to look for yourself at the discrepancies between the concerns raised by FDA scientists and the public FDA announcements, and do what you can to make *accurate* information immediately available to the more than 2 million women who have silicone breast implants, including the several hundred thousand who have the polyurethane covered devices.

In our conversation on Tuesday, you correctly identified restoring public confidence in FDA as a top priority. Dealing with the dangers of silicone breast implants in a more forthcoming manner could be an important step in that direction.

Sincerely,

TED WEISS
Chairman

* * * * *

TO: Ted Weiss, Chairman
FROM: Diana Zuckerman, Ph. D., Professional Staff Member
RE: PMA Applications for Silicone Breast Implants
DATE: September 12, 1991

In response to your request, I have conducted a preliminary review of the FDA premarket approval applications (PMAs) for breast implants that were submitted by Dow Corning, McGhan, Mentor, and Bioplasty (MISTI model). FDA has accepted all these applications for filing, which means they can remain on the market while FDA conducts a more thorough review during the approximately next five months.

FDA's decision to file these applications appears to be contrary to the recommendations made by the FDA statisticians, biologists, and other scientific experts, who consistently criticized the PMA studies for their major methodological flaws. *FDA scientists concluded that the studies of women with implants that were submitted by the companies were inadequate to provide evidence of safety or efficacy.* Although breast prostheses are intended for use over many years, FDA reviewers noted that there was almost no information about the experience of women who had implants for more than a few months. This is surprising, given that more than 2 million American women have breast implants, many for more than 10 years...

Dow Corning. In an August 12 memo to the file, the Task Leader of the FDA Breast Prosthesis PMA Task Force wrote that the Dow Corning clinical studies are "so weak that they cannot provide a reasonable assurance of the safety and effectiveness of these devices" because they provide "no assurance that the full range of complications are included, no dependable measure of the incidences of complications, no reliable measure of the revision rate and no quantitative measure of patient benefit." In his detailed criticism, he specified that the physicians who conducted the research were instructed "to report only complications associated with the implant. As a result the only complications reported are those at the implant site. This prevents these investigations from detecting systemic adverse effects or complications resulting [from] implantation of the devices." He also stated this "causes an underestimate of both the types and incidence of complications." Furthermore, each patient was examined only once after surgery and the number of patients examined at each time point is very small" making it difficult to determine the rate of complications at any point in time.

McGhan. The statistician who reviewed the McGhan PMA pointed out many major problems in their studies of women. For example, in the McGhan prospective clinical study, 10% of the 318 patients were not evaluated at the time they were discharged, and only one-third of the implants were assessed at the second required visit (3-6 months). The statistician pointed out that this lack of follow-up makes it impossible to draw any conclusions about long-term safety or effectiveness. . . . The statistician reported that the company's "historical cohort study" suffered from "strong potential for bias" and was therefore of no use in providing support for safety or effectiveness. An FDA biologist pointed out that the company studied only two of the four models listed on the PMA. This obviously makes it impossible to determine safety or effectiveness for the two "multilumen" models (made from saline and silicone) that were not studied. Moreover, only 39 reconstruction patients and 101 augmentation patients were studied, which isn't enough to determine problems (even fatal ones) that affect a small percentage of patients. In addition, many potential medical problems, such as breast disease or carcinoma, were not evaluated for all patients. My review of that PMA indicates that two-thirds of the women included in that study had prostheses implanted in 1989 or 1990; therefore, the study could not under any circumstances assess long-term risks.

Bioplasty. Similarly, a statistician reported that in the study of 860 patients with Bioplasty's MISTI Single or Double lumen implants, only 6% of the patients were assessed at the 2 year follow-up, and yet the company calculated their claims of safety and effectiveness as if they had followed large numbers of patients for two years . . . Most importantly, *the company stated that the physicians conducting the study refused to allow the company to contact the patients to ask about autoimmune disorders or cancer, "fearing that it may cause undue concern or violate patient confidentiality."* The company blamed the media, saying it "created an environment in which gathering that information was, at best, difficult."

Mentor. There were three PMAs submitted by Mentor, for three different types of implants. This in itself is interesting, since most companies submitted one PMA for several types of implants. The studies for the three types of implants were identical, and the statistician criticized the applications for failing to include important information, such as when patients were assessed subsequent to surgery, or whether appropriate steps were taken to avoid bias in the study. My review of the application reveals that the 806 patients in one study were apparently evaluated on the basis of the medical records, which did not necessarily provide any long-term information. For a second study, 128 of those 806 patients were interviewed on the telephone to evaluate their satisfaction with the implants. The 128 women represent 27% of the patients who were selected for the interview; it is therefore impossible to draw any conclusions about patient satisfaction based on that sample. In a third study by Mentor, 273 augmentation patients were included in a retrospective study about complications, but the information available was for an unspecified time, and based on available medical records of the plastic surgeon. Since such records would not be expected to include information on autoimmune disease or cancer, this study is inadequate in the safety information it can provide.

Conclusions. It is hard to understand why the companies, which have known since at least 1982 that they would probably be required to provide safety data, and which were warned more than three years ago that data would definitely be required, waited so long before they started conducting major studies. In fact, many of the studies were started in 1990 or 1991. Although prospective studies that followed women for many years would have been considered ideal, a reasonable alternative would be to start a study in 1990 that asked patients from the 1970's or early 1980's about any medical problems they have had since their implant surgery. That kind of thorough retrospective study was not conducted by any of the manufacturers.

In summary, there are several major problems with most of the studies:

1) Most do not study women for more than two years at the most; this is not sufficient to evaluate the safety of a medical device that is meant to be permanent, especially when the allegations have been made that they are likely to rupture after several years.

2) In many cases, the majority of women are lost to the study after a few months; it is therefore impossible to say whether an implant is safe if there is no information at all on most of the women who had the surgery.

3) In several studies, there are no relevant questions regarding autoimmune disorders, cancer, or other possible risks that have been associated with implants. It is not enough to look at medical records kept by plastic surgeons, since women will only return to their plastic surgeons for complications that they recognize to be associated with the surgery.

4) The number of reconstruction patients in most of the studies is so small, that they could not provide persuasive evidence of safety. Robert Sheridan informed me that for the purposes of filing, FDA assumed that the experiences of augmentation patients would be the same as those for reconstruction patients. That assumption is impossible to defend, since there are no data to back it up.

5) Several manufacturers have no studies of women with certain models of implants that they sell, or they have studied fewer than 10 women with particular types of implants. Again, Robert Sheridan told me that for the purposes of filing, the assumption was made that the safety of one model was the same as for other models. Again, that assumption is impossible to defend, since there are no data to back it up.

It will take years to provide meaningful long-term safety and to determine the average lifetime of breast prostheses that have been implanted in women. In some cases, well-designed studies are planned but have not yet been started.

*   *   *   *   *

September 13, 1991

David A. Kessler, M.D.
Commissioner
Food and Drug Administration
Rockville, MD 20857

Dear Dr. Kessler:

Last month, FDA announced that the premarket approval applications (PMAs) submitted by Dow Corning, McGhan, Mentor, and Bioplasty (MISTI model) have been accepted for filing. As a result of this decision, implants made by these manufacturers can remain on the market pending the full FDA review of the PMA applications. I am writing to urge your *immediate* review of these PMAs.

According to the reviews conducted by FDA statisticians, biologists, and other scientific experts, the decision to file seven PMAs appears to have virtually no support among FDA's scientific staff. *FDA's own scientists concluded that the studies of women with implants that were submitted by the companies were inadequate to provide evidence of safety or efficacy.*

Although breast prostheses are intended for use over many years, FDA reviewers noted that there was almost no information about the experiences of women who had implants for more than a few months. Despite FDA's requirement that they study the potential risks of autoimmune disease and cancer over long periods of time, the accepted PMAs contain virtually no information on these risks.

When new drugs or devices are introduced onto the market, the number of patients evaluated is necessarily small. However, in the case of breast implants, there is a 30 year history involving more than 2 million American women. There is no reason why the companies should not be held responsible for conducting thorough, unbiased research on large numbers of women to evaluate long-term safety and to determine the average lifetime of the implants.

It may be that FDA will eventually conclude that the statisticians and other scientists were correct, and reject all the PMA applications. Presumably, breast implants will then be removed from the market, except for research purposes, until adequate safety data are available. However, in the meantime, approximately 100,000 more American women may have prostheses implanted, not knowing that they are serving as guinea pigs in a vast, uncontrolled clinical trial.

None of the reviews and related FDA documents regarding the PMAs that have been provided to the subcommittee includes any justifications for filing the seven PMAs. Since I have been assured by FDA that the subcommittee has received all documents on this matter, I have to assume that there are no further FDA documents supporting the filing of any PMAs for breast implants. According to the attached review compiled by subcommittee staff, the main reasons for filing given by FDA officials were FDA's concern about a lengthy and unsuccessful appeals process, and concerns that the companies would not provide better safety information that could be made available to the public if the PMAs were not filed. I must question if these reasons represent an adequate regulatory test, or would even justify the amount of work that will be required of FDA staff to now fully evaluate applications that they have already determined to be hopelessly inadequate.

Because of the large number of letters that I have received from women with autoimmune diseases and other major illnesses that appear to be caused by ruptured implants, and the large number of women who would be expected to undergo surgery to implant prostheses during the months while FDA is determining whether to approve the seven PMAs, I am sending you this staff review and urging you to conduct an expedited review of all breast implant PMAs that have been filed.

In addition, kindly provide any other written documentation or explanations detailing the decision to accept the seven PMAs in light of the criticisms provided by your own scientific staff.

Sincerely,

TED WEISS
Chairman

*   *   *   *   *

Statement on Silicone Gel Breast Implants

by

David A. Kessler, M.D.

Commissioner of Food and Drugs

Washington, D.C.

January 6, 1992

Last November, an FDA advisory panel of outside experts agreed with our evaluation that the data supplied by the manufacturers were insufficient to establish that the implants are safe and effective.

Let me recap for you the original concerns about the gel implants that we brought to the advisory panel last November and that remain unanswered:

- We still do not know how often the implants leak, and when they do, we do not know exactly what materials get into the body.

- We still do not know how often the implants break, or how long they last.

- We still do not know how often women with the implants suffer adverse effects. For example, there are reports that painful hardening of the implant can occur in anywhere from 10 percent to 70 percent of patients.

- We still do not know to what extent the implants interfere with mammography examinations. This is especially important because the implants have been used in thousands of healthy women each year.

- We still do not know whether the implants can increase a

woman's risk of developing cancer.

- And we still do not know enough about the relationship between these devices and autoimmune and connective tissue diseases.

Thirty years of use and we still don't know the answers to these questions. Part of the problem is that, until 1976, there was no medical device law.

If you are not experiencing any difficulties, there is no need to consider removing the implants. However, if you are having symptoms you think may be related to your implants, you should see your doctor.

And all women with implants should have periodic check-ups for such problems as rupture. . . .

I want to stress that the FDA is not opposed to breast implants. We recognize the value of these devices, particularly for women who face a devastating and potentially disfiguring disease such as breast cancer.

We *want* to see safe breast implants available for all women who need them. But the manufacturers of silicone gel implants have failed thus far to provide adequate evidence that they are marketing a safe product.

We owe it to the American public to see to it that these questions are thoroughly investigated.

WOMEN FIND IT DIFFICULT TO GET BREAST IMPLANTS REMOVED

by Joan E. Rigdon

Staff Reporter
The Wall Street Journal
March 20, 1992

When Cynthia K. Buford decided to enlarge her breasts with silicone-gel implants in 1983, her doctor quickly scheduled surgery and billed her insurance.

But when she decided to get the implants removed after black goo began leaking from her nipples recently, Ms. Buford got a rude shock. Plastic surgeons, demanding cash up front, issued stern warnings about potential disfigurement.

One doctor told her to imagine "a very huge fat lady and look at the skin under her arms. That would give her an idea of what her breasts would look like if she didn't replace the implants after removing them, Ms. Buford recalls. "I came home and cried for three weeks."

In the end, she sought help at a county hospital, which demanded a down payment of $525 on a charge card. The total bill: more than $4,000.

Women are finding that it was much easier to get implants than it is to get rid of them. While Esther Rome, a member of the Boston Women's Health Book Collective, says, "It's impossible to document" the scarcity of doctors willing to remove implants, she adds that "it seems fairly widespread."

Getting the procedure performed is also emotionally draining. Many plastic surgeons predict deformity or encourage women to get replacement implants even if they don't want them. Most also say the procedure isn't medically necessary, so insurance companies are refusing to pay for it. (Some women have persuaded their insurers to pay by bypassing their surgeons and obtaining letters from family doctors and rheumatologists instead.)

Many plastic surgeons are reluctant because they fear lawsuits from other patients: removing implants is tantamount to admitting they're not safe. Critics charge that the implants can cause or trigger a variety of diseases, ranging from muscle pain to chronic immune disorders.

Even doctors who are willing to extract implants say they are being discouraged from doing so by insurers. One plastic surgeon says his insurance company, Doctor's Co. of Sonoma, Calif., advised him against performing a large number of removals. "They didn't want me to be a potentially higher risk person. . . . because it's such a lethal issue right now," the surgeon says. Dr. Mark Gorney, medical director of Doctor's Co., says that's "utter nonsense" and that removing implants isn't considered riskier than putting them in.

Removing implants can require more surgery than putting them in, because if the implants have ruptured, stray silicone must be scooped out. Polyurethane-covered implants can be especially difficult to remove if the polyurethane has mingled with scar tissue or surrounding muscle tissue.

Women's health groups have been steering women toward a few surgeons who also remove and study scar tissue to see if it has reacted with the silicone. One such surgeon, Dr. Lu-Jean Feng of Cleveland, has performed almost 100 implant removals on women from all over the U.S. But Ms. Rome of the Women's Health Book Collective says that so far she has searched unsuccessfully for a plastic surgeon in the Boston area who will remove and study scar tissue along with implants or send the tissue and implants to other researchers.

Some surgeons may be reluctant to remove implants for fear they will anger their colleagues or hurt their practices. One Texas woman, who traveled to Florida to have her implants removed in 1990, says her plastic surgeon told her he didn't want to remove too many implants in too short a time because "that would imply there was something wrong with them." The woman, a medical records worker, declined to be named.

. . . for many women, the quest for removal has become an odyssey. Ms. Buford, whose gel implants were covered with polyurethane foam, says she decided to have them removed after she developed knots in her breasts and "black stuff" began leaking from her nipples. The first plastic surgeon she consulted encouraged her to get replacements.

A second surgeon, Dr. Richard Burkett of Dallas, "told me I would want another set because I was going to look so disfigured" without implants. After comparing the likely result to a fat lady's arms, Dr. Burkett called her at home to repeat his warning that "I would not look right" without implants, Ms. Buford says. Dr. Burkett declined to return several phone calls seeking comment.

Devastated, Ms. Buford waited weeks before consulting another plastic surgeon, Dr. Diane Gibby of Dallas, who told her that surgery would make her flat-chested, not disfigured. "She's the one who started making me feel good about myself again," Ms. Buford says.

Patti Scher, a former nursing director who lives in Charlotte, N.C., flew with her husband to Cleveland so she could be operated on by Dr. Feng. Ms. Scher says that before her implants were removed, she suffered fatigue, blurred vision and night sweats that made her so weak she had to quit her job.

A NOTICE FROM THE ASPRS

by Norman Cole, MD
President, ASPRS
Letter to Commissioner Kessler, FDA
Feb. 19, 1992

In light of testimony that some physicians are refusing to see certain breast-implant patients, I would like to inform you that the American Society of Plastic and Reconstructive Surgeons recently initiated a national network of plastic surgeons who have agreed to counsel these women as a "safety net." This network can be easily accessed by calling the Society's toll-free "hotline," (800) 635-0635.

DOW CORNING CORPORATION PRESS CONFERENCE

Keith McKennon's Remarks

Thursday, March 19, 1992

The February FDA panel agreed that insufficient evidence exists to show any link between implants and systemic diseases of the immune system. The panel also said there is insufficient evidence to prove no such link exists. . . .

The FDA's current position, and the Advisory Panel's recommendation is that implants performing satisfactorily NEED NOT BE REMOVED. . . .

Dow Corning already has a replacement warranty program. This program, under appropriate circumstances, provides women using Dow Corning Silastic(R)II or MSI(R) Implants a replacement device and six hundred dollars in financial support. Dow Corning will continue that program, perhaps by increasing the dollar amount so that patients can purchase a device from other manufacturers.

The new program I am announcing today will be limited to patients with Dow Corning implants who have agreed with their physicians that, for medical reasons, their implant(s) need be removed, but who cannot afford the procedure. For such patients, we will provide up to $1,200 to support medical costs of the removal procedure. Patients in the USA can call Dow Corning's Breast Implant Information Center to find out more information about the program.

This program will be available throughout the USA, and we

are reviewing the need for such programs in other parts of the world. . . .

We have decided that Dow Corning will not resume the production or sales of breast implants. . . .

Our reasons for not resuming production and sales . . . are not related to issues of science or safety but to the existing condition of the marketplace. . . .

The products represent less than 1% of our revenues and have not been profitable over their history. Given the continued controversial environment surrounding this product, I see no prospect for business improving. Instead, it seems likely that the future use of this product will be curtailed to a considerable extent. . . .

Let me close by assuring women who have our implants that we remain fully committed to them as the manufacturer of their device—we will stand by them, by our commitments to continuing research, and by our other support programs. . . .

For more information, patients can call Dow Corning's Breast Implant Information Center at (800) 442-5442. [Physicians should call (800) 437-7056.]

What should I do if my Dow Corning implants need replacement?

. . . women will be able to obtain replacement breast implants from other manufacturers.

What impact will this issue have on other silicone medical products manufactured and supplied by Dow Corning?

The properties and performance of silicones as a biomaterial have been demonstrated to be extremely effective and are integral to modern medical technology.

Silicones used in medical devices and pharmaceutical products are produced in three primary forms: liquid, gel and elastomer, a solid form of silicone. Our primary participation is through the sale of materials to people who manufacture medical devices and pharmaceutical products. Through our subsidiary, Dow Corning Wright, we also selectively produce, market and sell finished products, the vast majority of which are in the form of molded, cured elastomeric products used by physicians and other medical professionals. Examples include finger joints, catheters, intravenous tubing systems and the hydrocephalus shunt . . .

[Editor's note: Dow Corning Wright is in the process of removing all of its silicone products for cosmetic surgery from the market—KO]

DOW CORNING PREPARES FOR FLOOD OF LAWSUITS OVER BREAST IMPLANTS

By Susan Moffat

Los Angeles Times
March 13, 1992

Facing hundreds of lawsuits and threats of thousands more over its breast implants, Dow Corning is girding itself to handle financial liabilities of still unknown proportions and taking measures to protect its hugely successful business of supplying silicone to industries including aerospace, automobiles and computers.

The company is appealing a recent jury verdict of $7.3 million in damages by a woman who said her implants caused connective tissue disease, and it argues vigorously that it has no liability in the case.

So far, Dow Corning is saying it doesn't expect lawsuits to be a threat to the company. The company said recently that it has $250 million in insurance to cover possible claims. Lawrence Reed, Dow Corning's chief operating officer, earlier said, "We believe we have reserves adequate for what we know today." The company already announced that it has set aside $25 million to handle costs of shutting down its breast implant manufacturing business in the fourth quarter of 1991.

But J. Douglas Peters, a Detroit attorney who has filed a

number of suits against Dow Corning, said he figures that the company's eventual liability could run from $1 billion to $2 billion.

Peters and many plaintiffs' lawyers argue that the company may be in no rush to settle lawsuits, waiting instead for cases to accumulate so that it can make a case for a Chapter 11 bankruptcy filing—a process that could mitigate the ultimate payout and might not necessarily be disruptive to the company. Reed countered that the company is "absolutely not thinking in terms of bankruptcy" and said the bulk of the company's product lines are going strong.

Peters noted that in another case involving a medical device, A. H. Robins, maker of the Dalkon Shield intrauterine contraceptive, filed for bankruptcy protection in 1985 after lawsuits by women and their families who said the IUDs caused infertility, miscarriages and even death.

A. H. Robins sought protection when liability from hundreds of thousands of claims from women exceeded its assets. Under Chapter 11 bankruptcy protection, the company set aside $2.4 billion to settle the suits, and sold itself to giant American Home Products in 1989 in a $700-million stock swap. Many women who had the devices complain that the bankruptcy settlement unfairly limited their compensation, despite the fact that the restructured company enjoys strong sales of such popular products as Chap Stick and Robitussin cough syrup.

As of mid-February, Dow Corning said about 200 lawsuits relating to its breast implants had been filed. But more are being filed daily, and some lawyers are predicting that tens of thousands may be filed by some of the estimated 1 million to 2 million women who have breast implants made by various manufacturers, including Bioplasty, Mentor, and McGhan.

Dow Corning may be liable for injuries caused by other makers' implants because they supply the silicone gel that fills many of them, plaintiffs' lawyers said.

Sal Liccardo, a San Jose lawyer, has filed about 110 suits against Dow Corning and other implant makers, is preparing about a hundred more and is getting 15 to 30 calls a day from women who say they have health problems related to the implants.

Peters said his firm is preparing more than 150 cases after about 400 phone calls from women with implants. He expects damage awards of about $500,000 for each plaintiff, and, he said, there may be well over 20,000 lawsuits. About 700,000 women have implants made by Dow Corning, Peters said. It could take six to 10 years of litigation before women can collect any money, he said.

Dow Corning is a 50-50 joint venture of Dow Chemical and Corning Inc. Both companies said they have no liability because Dow Corning is independently managed. But some lawyers believe that suits could reach as far as the parent companies, especially if Dow Corning runs out of assets to handle the suits. Corning, which relies on Dow Corning for about a quarter of its earnings and saw its share price plummet after press attention to the breast implant problems, is facing 10 shareholder suits charging that it did not reveal negative information on the silicone company. The company denies the charges and says problems at Dow Corning will have "no significant impact" on Corning's earnings in 1992.

SILICONE IMPLANTS AVAILABLE ONLY FOR STUDY PURPOSES

HHS NEWS

U.S. Department of Health and Human Services

April 16, 1992

The Food and Drug Administration today announced that silicone breast implants will be available only under controlled clinical studies. Women who need these implants for reconstruction will be assured access to those studies. . . .

"Some women need these implants for . . . certain congenital disorders," said Dr. Kessler. "While this policy is meant to be compassionate toward these patients, it is not to be interpreted as *'business as usual.'* Our primary goal is to put in place a process to obtain adequate information about the safety of these devices. . . ."

Further tightly controlled research studies will be set up to obtain more information on safety and effectiveness. They will allow limited availability for women desiring the implants for augmentation . . . Manufacturers will be required to conduct a separate study for each model of implant they wish to market. The studies will focus on specific safety questions about the implants. . . .

The studies will help answer questions about side effects, such as capsular contracture, calcium deposits, interference with mammography readings, implant leakage or rupture and changes in the sensation of the breasts.

Questions about possible long-term effects such as immune-related disorders and cancer will be answered by epidemiological studies of women who already have implants. . . .

FDA will also require laboratory studies to be conducted by the manufacturers, under a strict time table, to look at the chemical composition and toxicity of the silicone material that "bleeds" out of the implant shell, the strength of the implant shell, its resistance to rupture and the physical and chemical changes that the implants may undergo in the body.

FDA has established a toll-free telephone line to provide information materials to consumers on breast implants. The number is (800) 532-4440.

PUBLIC CITIZEN RESPONDS TO EXPERIMENTAL IMPLANTS

STATEMENT BY
SIDNEY M. WOLFE, M.D.
Director, Public Citizen Health Research Group
In response to FDA announcement about
experimental use of silicone gel
April 16, 1992

. . . Even though FDA should not have authorized this unprecedented human experiment, the overwhelming majority of women will choose not to have silicone gel breast implants, devices whose future is likely to be finished. . . .

A March 30th draft of the informed consent sheet which would be used by all women getting implants for reconstruction or augmentation lists seven "known risks" of breast implants:

- capsular contracture (which can cause "unnatural firmness, pain and, in severe cases, a misshapen appearance");

- calcium deposits in the tissue around the implant;

- granulomas or "non-cancerous lumps" "which may be difficult to distinguish . . . from cancerous lumps;"

- gel "bleed" and rupture of the implant with migration;

- interference with mammography;

- changes in nipple and breast sensation;

- interference with breast feeding.

Many of the plastic surgeons who have already switched to saline implants because of the moratorium are not likely to switch back to this more dangerous alternative. The main group of women who will still choose to have silicone gel breast implants are those whose surgeons will continue, as they have in the past, to lie about the risks of these devices and thereby "override" the strong warnings in the informed consent sheet.

We continue to recommend that women not get silicone gel implants.

NATIONWIDE SURVEY OF WOMEN WITH BREAST IMPLANTS FOR AUGMENTATION

Projected by Public Citizen Health Research Group to all U.S. women (1.495 million) with breast implants for augmentation. Based on a survey of 100,000 American households "chosen to represent the nation's consumer population," funded by the American Society of Plastic and Reconstructive Surgeons

Type of Complications	% in survey with problem	projected # of women with problem*
Complications such as rupture or infection	5% of women	75,000 women
Hard breasts	5% of women	75,000 women
Breast firmness: somewhat or very bothersome	11.4% of women	171,000 women
Scars somewhat or very visible	30% of women	449,000 women
Breasts somewhat or very unnatural/ uncomfortable	7% of women	105,000 women
Bothersome changes in nipple sensation	12.4% of women	185,000 women
Pain and sensitivity complaints	5% of women	75,000 women

PUBLIC CITIZEN ANSWERS TO QUESTIONS ABOUT SILICONE GEL BREAST IMPLANTS

by Public Citizen Health Research Group

Q. I have implants and have had no problems. Should I have them removed?

A. We do not recommend removal of non-problematic implants.

. . .

The following physical symptoms may indicate a problem with your implants: *pain or hardening of your breasts, rashes, extreme fatigue, fevers, joint and/or muscle pain, burning or "electric" sensation, skin "thickening" or skin hardening.* If you experience these or other prolonged, unexplained or undiagnosed physical symptoms, consult your surgeon; there may be a problem with your implants. You may also wish to consult a rheumatologist or internist.

Q. How can I tell if my implant has ruptured? If it has ruptured, should it be removed?

A. In addition to manual examination and mammography, the physical symptoms that are described in question 1 can also apply to implant rupture. If you have experienced any trauma to the chest, this too can cause implant rupture. You may also notice a difference in size or feel to a breast with a ruptured implant.

It may be easier to determine implant rupture by having a mammogram. This procedure can detect most ruptures and residual silicone. Ruptured implants should be removed.

Q. If an implant is removed, should the scar tissue "capsule" also be removed?

A. Yes. If an implant has ruptured, most of the silicone will migrate to the surrounding tissues and lymph nodes. It is best to remove as much of the silicone gel as possible, thus lessening the likelihood of complications.

Q. I went to my doctor, and he/she assured me that my implants are intact, not ruptured. I am still having some physical problems. How can this be explained?

A. Even an intact implant has a normal amount of "gel bleed." This microscopic amount of silicone gel that bleeds through the outer envelope of the implant can be enough to cause the symptoms discussed above. Also note that ruptures can be missed by even the best mammograms.

Q. My implants have hardened, and my surgeon has told me it is a "simple office procedure" to break the scar tissue. What is this and should I agree to it?

A. Your surgeon is referring to a "closed capsulotomy." When breasts become hard, this is because scar tissue has formed around the implant. Breaking up the scar tissue will make the breast soft again; however, accomplishing this by closed capsulotomy (manual pressure on the breast) may cause the implant to tear or rupture. While this procedure may seem simpler than an "open capsulotomy" (a surgical procedure), the risks of implant rupture are great. Although for 20 years, plastic surgeons were advised and taught how to do this procedure, the manufacturers' most recent package inserts caution surgeons *not* to perform closed capsulotomies because of the high risk of rupture.

If your surgeon performs an open capsulotomy, it is recommended that old implants *not* be re-inserted, as there is a risk that the old implant could be damaged. Also be aware that your old implants are *your* property and you should keep them for examination by an independent lab for analysis. Your request to save your implants should be made, in writing, to your surgeon and hospital *before* your surgery.

Q. How long do silicone gel implants last?

A. Although originally promoted as a "once in a lifetime procedure," manufacturers are now acknowledging that this is not true. Actual "body life" of an implant is probably closer to 10 years. You should be aware that if you are considering this procedure, depending upon your age at time of implantation, you will probably need to undergo replacement surgery at some point in the future. You should also be aware that in the current package inserts for Dow implants, there is no mention of a time warranty.

Q. Why have the implants been on the market if they were not approved by the FDA?

A. Silicone gel-filled breast implants were on the U.S. market before the FDA received regulatory authority over medical devices in 1976. They were therefore "grandfathered" onto the market. The FDA, in 1991, required manufacturers who wished to continue marketing their implants to submit Pre-Market Approval (PMA) applications, thus initiating FDA review of safety and effectiveness data. . . .

BREAST AUGMENTATION
A RISK FACTOR FOR
BREAST CANCER?

By Hans Berkel, M.D., PhD.,
Dale C. Birdsell, M.D., and
Heather Jenkins

ABSTRACT *Background.* A relation between breast augmentation and the subsequent risk of breast cancer has been postulated. Since an estimated 2 million women in the United States alone have received breast implants, even a small increase in the risk of breast cancer could have considerable public health consequences.

Methods. We performed a population-based nonconcurrent cohort-linkage study. All women in Alberta, Canada, who underwent cosmetic breast augmentation from 1973 through 1986 were included in the implant cohort (n=11,676). This cohort was compared with the cohort of all women in Alberta in whom a first primary breast cancer was diagnosed (n=13,557). The expected number of breast-cancer cases in the implant cohort was estimated by applying age-specific and calendar-year-specific incidence rates of breast cancer (obtained from

Reprinted with permission from the *New England Journal of Medicine*, June 18, 1992. Copyright 1992, by the Massachusetts Medical Society.

the Alberta Cancer Registry) to the implant cohort. Standard-ized incidence ratios were calculated by dividing the observed by the expected number of breast-cancer cases in the implant cohort.

Results. Forty-one patients with implants were subsequently found to have breast cancer. The expected number was 86.2. The standardized incidence ratio was thus 47.6 percent, signifi-cantly lower than expected (P < 0.01). The average length of follow-up in the implant cohort was 10.2 years, and the average length of time from breast augmentation to the diagnosis of breast cancer was 7.5 years.

Conclusions. Women who undergo breast augmentation with silicone implants have a lower risk of breast cancer than the general population. This finding suggests that these women are drawn from a population already at low risk and that the implants do not substantially increase the risk.

Prosthetic breast augmentation and reconstruction have been practiced for several decades and have been considered to be safe and accepted surgical procedures. Smooth-walled silicone implants (filled with silicone gel or saline) have been the most common type of prosthesis used. Scar encapsulation of these implants frequently leads to compression and undesir-able firmness. To overcome these complications, implants cov-ered with polyurethane sponge were reintroduced in the 1980s in the United States and Canada. Recently, however, concern has been raised about the carcinogenic potential of the break-down products of polyurethane. The breakdown products (i.e., toluene 2,4-diisocyanate and toluene 2,6-diisocyanate diamines) were reportedly found in the urine of a patient with polyure-thane-sponge-covered implants. These substances are known to cause sarcomas in rats. An expert panel of the Canadian Medical Association concluded, however, that "surgical removal of polyurethane-foam-covered breast implants solely for reasons of potential risk of cancer does not appear to be indicated." Despite this statement there has been considerable public concern about the potentially increased risk of breast cancer after cosmetic breast augmentation. In the scientific literature few studies have addressed the issue. To our knowledge only four studies have been reported to date, and three of these consisted of surveys mailed to plastic surgeons. Although no excessive risk was found, the strength of the evidence in this type of study is limited because of the great potential for ascertainment and recall bias. In one epidemiologic study, no increased risk was found.

It is estimated that 2 million women in the United States have received breast implants. Thus, from a public health perspective it is important to determine the extent of any increase in risk in these women, even if it is only a small one. To evaluate the potential difference in the risk of breast cancer among women who have undergone breast augmentation, we decided to perform a nonconcurrent cohort-linkage study.

The original implant cohort consisted of 14,545 patients. A total of 2869 were excluded from further analysis for the reasons given in Table 1. The majority (60 percent) were excluded because they had duplicate records. In these cases the first year (and the records pertaining to that date) were retained in the data base. These women were included in further analyses. Also excluded from the implant cohort were 315 women who had received implants as part of reconstructive surgery after mastectomy for breast cancer. After these exclusions, the implant cohort consisted of 11,676 women. From the cancer registry data base we selected all the patients with first primary breast cancers diagnosed from 1973 through 1990. During these 18 years a total of 13,557 women in Alberta were given such a diagnosis. These women constituted the breast-cancer cohort. The cancer registry has a continuous quality-control monitoring program in place; therefore, we are confident that the data on breast-cancer cases from the registry are complete and valid.

Table 1. Reasons for Exclusion from the Implant Cohort of 14,545 Patients.

Reason for Exclusion	No. of Patients
Male Sex	218
Treated outside study period	102
Exceeded age limit	512
Duplicate record	1,722
Reconstructive Surgery	315
Total	2,869
Total after exclusions	11,676

Table 2 shows the age distribution of the two cohorts. As expected, the implant cohort was much younger: 86.0 percent of the women in this cohort were less than 40 years of age, whereas 91.6 percent of the women in the breast-cancer cohort were at least 40 years of age at the time of diagnosis.

Table 2. Age Distribution of the Women with Breast Implants and the Women with BreastCancer.

Age Group yr	Implant Cohort*	Breast-Cancer Cohort
	number (%)	
20-24	1,997 (17.1)	12 (0.1)
25-29	3,287 (28.2)	114 (0.8)
30-34	3,048 (26.1)	351 (2.6)
35-39	1,711 (14.6)	662 (4.9)
40-44	824 (7.1)	1,079 (8.0)
45-49	436 (3.7)	1,502 (11.1)
50-54	232 (2.0)	1,531 (11.3)
55-59	94 (0.8)	1,613 (11.9)
60-64	41 (0.4)	1,580 (11.6)
65 or over	—	5,113 (37.7)
Total	11,670	13,557

*Six women in the implant cohort were excluded because there was no evidence of breast augmentation.

The two cohorts were linked, and a total of 47 matching women were identified in whom breast augmentation preceded the diagnosis of breast cancer. The hospital charts of these women were reviewed, and in six of them no evidence of an implant procedure was found. Neither the medical history of the patient nor the mammograms revealed any evidence of breast augmentation. These six women were excluded from further analyses. The 41 women confirmed to have had implant procedures before cancer was diagnosed had bilateral augmentation. These 41 women constituted 0.4 percent of the original cohort of 11,670 women with implants.

The total number of person-years at risk for the women in the study was 124,494. The average follow-up was 10.2 years (range, 1 to 18); 58.1 percent of the cohort had at least 10 years of follow-up (Table 3). Only 29 of the women in the implant cohort (0.2 percent) were followed for less than five years.

A total of 86.2 cases of breast cancer were expected, and only 41 were observed. The standardized incidence ratio was thus 47.6 percent—significantly less than expected (P < 0.01) . . . In all age groups the standardized incidence ratios were significantly lower than expected; in fact, the ratios were remarkably constant across the age groups.

A short interval between the date of implantation and the date of diagnosis of the cancer could indicate that a tumor was present subclinically at the time of augmentation. We therefore determined the length of this interval for the 41 women; the average was 7.5 years. In 80 percent of the women (33 of 41), the implant procedure was performed at least five years before the diagnosis of the cancer. The interval between implantation and the diagnosis of breast cancer was at least 10 years in 11 cases (27 percent).

The mean age at implantation of the 41 women in whom

breast cancer later developed was 38.3 years (range, 20 to 64); the mean age at diagnosis was 45.7 years (range, 30 to 68).

DISCUSSION

Using the same design as in our study, Deapen et al. reported a standardized incidence ratio of 57 in a cohort of 3111 women who were followed for an average of 6.2 years. The average length of follow-up in our study was almost twice as long (10.2 years), and more than half of our cohort were followed for at least 10 years. The question arises, however, whether even this length of follow-up is adequate to allow a plausible lead time between exposure (implantation) and outcome (the diagnosis of breast cancer). To evaluate this problem, we excluded all women from the implant cohort for whom fewer than 10 years of follow-up data were available. This adjustment resulted in the exclusion of 4892 women. Applying the same methods as described earlier, we found that the expected number of cancer cases in the remaining 6778 women was 67.8. Eleven cases of breast cancer were observed. The standardized incidence ratio in this subcohort with a long follow-up was 16.2. Thus, in women with long-term follow-up after implantation (the average number of years of follow-up in this group was 13.3 years; range, 10 to 18), no increased risk of breast cancer was found.

The size of the cohort in our study was nearly four times that of the study by Deapen and colleagues (11,670 vs. 3111). In the latter the implant cohort consisted of patients treated by 35 plastic surgeons in Los Angeles; therefore, it was not a population-based study—a factor that could give rise to ascertainment bias. In our study all women who had breast augmentation in Alberta from 1973 through 1986 were included in the study and matched with patients from the population-based cancer registry. We believe that this makes ascertainment bias an unlikely explanation of our results.

Our study yielded a result similar to that of the study by

Deapen et al.: there was no increased risk of breast cancer after breast augmentation. In addition to these two cohort studies, the results of three surveys among plastic surgeons, inquiring about the frequency of cancers in women with implants, have been reported. Although the evidence in this type of study is not strong, these studies also did not indicate an increased frequency of breast cancer. Case reports do not allow an evaluation of the question of a difference in risk.

Could the result of our study be explained by the influence of bias? As mentioned, ascertainment bias is unlikely to explain the absence of an increased risk. The very nature of the nonconcurrent cohort-study design eliminates recall bias as a potential explanation. From the data on radiation risk, it appears that younger women are more sensitive to a radiation effect than older women. The question thus arises whether the age of women at implantation could be a confounding factor in the determination of the subsequent risk of breast cancer. By using age-specific and calendar year-specific incidence rates in calculating the expected number of cases of breast cancer, however, we have controlled for a potential age effect.

In the study by Deapen et al., a large number of patients were lost to follow-up (approximately 14 percent) because of the mobility of the California population and the difficulty of gaining access to out-of-state records. A study in Alberta of women with cervical cancer found that approximately 10 percent of the cohort moved out of the province. Nevertheless, women who were living in Alberta but whose cancers were diagnosed or treated in another province would also have been reported to the Alberta Cancer Registry. We believe that the loss to follow-up cannot explain the low standardized incidence ratios found in our study.

We found six false positive matches. In these cases, the wrong fee code was probably used or entered in the Alberta Department of Health data base. It is possible that there were also false negative "matches," resulting in a lower observed number and therefore in an artificially low standardized incidence ratio. However, since we allowed for logical errors in data entry during the linkage procedure, we do not believe that undermatching is a plausible explanation of the low number of breast cancer observed. To eliminate this possibility, we randomly selected a 1 percent sample of patients with breast cancer in the registry and reviewed their charts to evaluate whether there was any evidence of implantation. In all cases there was no indication of implantation either in the medical history or on the mammograms. We believe there is no possibility that false negative matches explain the results of our study.

Another possible explanation of the low standardized incidence ratio found in our study could be that cancer in women with implants is diagnosed at a later stage (i.e., it has not yet been discovered, thus lowering the number of observed cases). Preliminary results of a survival analysis of the group of women with implants who had cancer showed no difference in survival between these women and women without breast implants who had cancer. We therefore do not think that there is a substantially longer latency period in women with breast implants before a tumor is diagnosed.

Finally, one could hypothesize that women who undergo augmentation mammoplasty have a much lower a priori risk of breast cancer, which may or may not be affected by the presence of the implants. No information about the base-line risk of breast cancer or the prevalence of risk factors among women who have implants is available. Theoretically, therefore, one could argue that the results of our study do not permit the conclusion that implants do not increase the risk of breast cancer (because of the unknown base-line risk), despite the fact that any such risk does not reach that in the general population of women of comparable age during the same period. Strictly speaking, then, we have not ruled out the possibility that implants increase the risk of breast cancer in a highly selected group of women with a very low base-line risk. Women who undergo breast augmentation are in general of higher socioeconomic status (a factor that increases the risk of breast cancer). On the other hand, augmentation for cosmetic reasons is usually done in slim women with small breasts, and small breasts have been considered a favorable factor, lowering the risk. The relation between breast size and the risk of cancer is controversial, however.

This study focuses on women who had silicone implants for cosmetic breast augmentation. Approximately 85 percent of the women received smooth-walled implants filled with silicone gel, whereas the remainder received smooth-walled implants filled with saline. During the study period, prophylactic mastectomy followed by reconstructive surgery was very rarely done. Polyurethane-sponge-covered implants were not used in Alberta during the study period. It probably will not be possible to evaluate the effects of such implants for 5 to 10 years, at which time a sufficient number of person-years at risk will have been accumulated in women with this type of implant.

In summary, our study did not find an increased risk of cancer among women who had received breast implants, although the length of follow-up, the completeness of follow-up and the size of the cohort would have allowed the detection of such a risk. Questions that remain to be answered include what the risk estimates are for other cancers and what the survival experience is of women who had breast cancer after cosmetic breast augmentation.

[Editor's note: The study indicates that 86% of the women pulled up in the Alberta Department of Health computer were under 40 when they received their implants. How old are they now? What proportion of the women with implants are still under 40 years of age as of January 1, 1991?

40 is the age at which the incidence of breast cancer in women begins to increase. Therefore, one of the flaws of this study is that a disproportionately high percentage of its "participants" from the implant cohort appear to be in a known low risk group due to their age. Most women do not even begin getting regular mammograms until the age of 40 or older. The

data does not show how many have reached this age-related higher risk group, nor when, nor whether these women had the regular mammograms and breast checks recommended for women aged 40 and older.

The fine public health system and excellent record-keeping in Alberta notwithstanding, doctors would have no reason to search extra-diligently for breast cancer in women youger than 40. As the younger recipients of breast implants age, the data in this study may change.

Furthermore, no data regarding frequency or thoroughness of screening for breast cancer in any age group is indicated in the study.

None of these women were actually seen and evaluated in person. This information comes from a computer database, rather than existential reality, and the study may have been performed during the last few months, given its nonconcurrency. Who funded this study? A group of doctors, or a disinterested third party?

The actual number of women with breast implants who also have as yet undetected breast cancer may be quite different than appears in the data presented here. A more effective procedure would be to use the Alberta implant cohort and examine each woman for signs of cancer. And the study should not be limited to breast cancer but should show the incidence of all cancers in breast augmentation patients. Such a study would be costly and time-consuming.

The statement that "women who undergo breast augmentation with silicone implants have a lower risk of breast cancer than the general population" seems very irresponsible. Breast augmentation should not be perceived by anyone as a preventative measure for breast cancer—KO]

THE SILICONE CONTROVERSY
WHEN WILL SCIENCE PREVAIL?

by Jack C. Fisher, MD

The fate of the silicone-gel breast implant may have been foretold in 1988 when a member of the Food and Drug Administration's advisory panel on general and plastic surgical devices suggested that because the benefits of breast implants were unclear, their use should not be allowed if there was any associated risk. Several members of the advisory panel and the FDA have recently displayed similar insensitivity to the demonstrated needs of more than a million women who since 1963 have sought breast implantation for cosmetic or reconstructive purposes.

The attitude of the FDA and its actions this past year have depended largely on the exaggerated claims of consumer-advocacy groups and on poorly documented assertions. And there are indications that the FDA's approach will extend to other silicone medical products as well.

Meanwhile, the carefully considered position statements of many respected organizations—including the American Medical Association, American College of Surgeons, American College of Radiology, American College of Rheumatology, Society of

Reprinted with permission from the *New England Journal of Medicine,* June 18, 1992. Copyright 1992, by the Massachusetts Medical Society.

Surgical Oncologists, and American Society of Plastic and Re-constructive Surgeons—seem to have been ignored by the FDA. These and other responsible professional organizations have sought to place the risks of silicone implantation in perspective with respect to the benefits derived, but with little success.

Silicone (polydimethylsiloxane) was first used clinically in liquid form during World War II, when glass syringes were lubricated with silicone so that they would function reliably in combat. Silicone is an inorganic polymer of silicone dioxide with elastomeric properties. It exists in liquid, gel, or solid form.

Today, the many hundreds of uses of this material inside and outside the body have spawned a major industry in silicone medical products, still largely American. The administration of drugs and parenteral fluids, as well as hemodialysis and cardiac-bypass technology, depends on liquid silicone. Over time, patients with insulin-dependent diabetes and those who depend on dialysis accumulate substantial bodily exposure to silicone. Yet no systemic illness attributable to silicone had been reported in diabetics or in patients undergoing long-term hemodialysis.

Not until 1976 was the oversight of devices added to the responsibilities of the FDA. Twelve years later, the silicone-gel breast implant entered what has become a very troubled period of evaluation. The saline-filled silicone-shell breast implant is not yet affected by the FDA's restrictions, but will come under review later this year.

Silicone, like all foreign materials placed within planes of tissue, produces a fibrous reaction, often called a capsule when it surrounds a breast implant. Contraction of the capsule and compression of a pliable gel implant can lead to breast firm-ness. The frequency of the resultant contractures is a subjective determination based on patients' acceptance and surgeons' standards. A survey of patients conducted by the American Society of Plastic Surgery in 1990 showed contractures in 26 percent of the patients who received implants for cosmetic augmentation and 38 percent of those who received implants for reconstruction after mastectomy. Few patients, however, had considered removal of the implant, and fewer still had acted on their dissatisfaction.

Concern about an increased risk of breast cancer after silicone implantation has been expressed repeatedly by Dr. Sidney Wolfe of the advocacy group Public Citizen, most recently at the February 1992 FDA hearing on silicone-gel breast implants. The only cancers ever plausibly attributed to silicone, however, were connective-tissue sarcomas that appeared in strains of rodents susceptible to cancer—a phenomenon known as solid-state carcinogenesis. Silicone has not been known to cause breast cancer in any animal species. Human sarcomas caused by implantable materials are rare and are more likely to be associated with metallic implants. Implanted silicone has not to my knowledge been associated with human sarcoma.

Epidemiologic studies have been conducted in Los Angeles and in Alberta, Canada; neither identified any increase in breast cancer among women with breast implants as compared with those without. A third study is in progress, and a fourth will soon be funded by the National Cancer Institute.

Silverstein et al. have called attention to the potential for delayed diagnosis of breast cancer in women with breast implants. No such delay has yet been confirmed. However, breast implants of any composition can impede the interpretation of mammograms, more because of the compression of breast tissue than because of the opacity of the implant. Nevertheless, the American College of Radiology believes that an adequate examination can be achieved with commonly available techniques, and it does not support restricting the use of breast implants.

Speculation that connective-tissue diseases may result from silicone breast implantation has persisted without substantiation since 1982. The American College of Rheumatology recently issued its own statement: "There is no convincing evidence that these implants cause any generalized disease." Additional investigation is encouraged because of continuing reports of musculoskeletal symptoms in some women with breast implants. These have largely been individual case reports, most without adequate laborative study, clinical documentation, or follow-up. Weisman et al. conducted the only quantitative study that has used epidemiologic methods, but they could not identify any cause-and-effect relation between breast implants and rheumatic disease.

What is the likelihood that silicone might cause an autoimmune disorder? Immunologists doubt that it could serve as an antigen by itself, and no evidence suggests that it does. Heggers has identified antibodies to silicon-protein complexes, but the finding is not specific to breast implants and the antibodies cannot be correlated with rheumatic disease. They may be natural antibodies and are probably not indicative of autoimmune disease. No convincing evidence shows that the removal of breast implants reverses the musculoskeletal symptoms attributed to their implantation.

It would in fact be difficult to protect anyone in a developed society from biologic exposure to silicone. The material is widely used in food, beverage, and cosmetics industries. We consume and inspire microdroplets of silicone. Consider a patient with longstanding insulin-dependent diabetes, who may over time inject 25,000 to 50,000 microdroplets (25 to 50 g) of silicone with a cumulative surface area larger than that of any implantable device now in use (unpublished data).

Serious medical sequelae aside, concern has also been expressed about the durability and life span of the breast implant. The saline inflatable silicone implant can deflate (an incidence of 1 to 5 percent has been reported), usually requiring replacement. What about the silicone-gel implant?

The outer shell, or envelope, of the gel is a semipermeable membrane through which microdroplets are known to pass. Gel penetration, or "bleed," as it has come to be known, is microscopic, involving the dispersal of only a few grams in a typical fibrous capsule. Scanning electron microscopy shows 1 to 2 mm of penetration. The spreading inkblot of silicone that has been depicted in television graphics is simply not accurate. Silicone is hydrophobic, and as microdroplets it does not migrate easily through an aquaeous environment. Macrodroplets of silicone injected by needle may have sufficient mass to migrate according to gravitational force. The only other way for silicone to move in the body is for microscopic droplets or particles to be picked by macrophages. Silicone has occasionally been identified in lymph nodes after breast or orthopedic implantation.

The penetration of silicone gel has not been correlated with postoperative breast firmness. Since 1980 a barrier coat in the envelope of all silicone-gel implants has sharply reduced gel penetration.

Rupture is another concern, one that has been overstated and confused in the press. The word "rupture" can be applied to the implant envelope or to the fibrous capsule that surrounds the implant. A mammogram can reveal a capsular rupture but not necessarily the failure of an implant envelope. The possibility of silent rupture—a failed implant in an intact fibrous capsule—therefore exists. In such cases the patient is entirely asymptomatic and the mammogram is normal.

Symptomatic or extracapsular rupture of a gel implant has been uncommon in 30 years of experience with the devices. Rupture suggested by physical signs or confirmed by breast imaging requires the replacement of the implant. Nevertheless, no systemic medical illnesses have been attributed to either symptomatic or silent rupture.

David Kessler, the head of the FDA, has said that we know more about the life of an automobile tire than about that of a breast implant. But unlike tires, implantable devices are out of sight and serve their function until clinical evidence suggests otherwise. One reason why we do not know more about the durability of implants is because failure has been uncommon, and in the absence of reliable imaging methods, surgical exploration of asymptomatic women cannot be justified.

The worries prompted by the efforts of Public Citizen, the FDA, and the press have caused many patients without symptoms to ask that their implants be removed or exchanged, a process that offers some opportunity to define the rate of implant failure. But reports of failure are influenced by new variables that confound interpretation. For example, the current role of plaintiffs' attorneys in decisions to remove implants creates monetary incentives to identify defective implants at the time of removal. After the moratorium on the use of breast implants was announced by Dr. Kessler on January 6, 1992, a torrent of legal activity began. The American Trial Lawyers Association conducts regular seminars for plaintiffs' attorneys, assisted by selected data provided by Dr. Wolfe of Public Citizen, an organization that conducts no scientific research of its own, yet offers scientific judgments.

Only two manufacturers of silicone breast implants remain in the American market. Expansion and development have moved to Europe, where review of the same evidence has produced conclusions contrary to those of the FDA. There are 1600 manufacturers of silicone medical products in the United States, and many feel that legal precedents unleashed by the FDA's handling of the breast-implant issue will soon affect their market. The price of silicone medical products, 30 to 40 percent of which goes toward legal defense and obtaining regulatory approval, has already been affected.

In the midst of this controversy, what are women with implants thinking? Many are frightened, despite the absence of documented problems. A few, angered by what they believe to be insufficient forewarning, have joined together. Their voices, although not numerous, are easily heard in today's media-oriented society. Many of these women have suffered, but not necessarily from any biologic effect of implanted silicone. Some are simply victims of bad surgery.

Most of the 1 percent of American women who have opted for breast implants have been reassured and go on with their lives. Fortunately, the FDA has been careful not to recommend any mass removal of breast implants. But the impact of the FDA's current position will be harshest on women who for their own reasons want breast reconstruction or cosmetic surgery in the future and who will now be subject to the agency's complex guidelines.

BREAST IMPLANTS
PROTECTION OR
PATERNALISM?

by Marcia Angell, MD

In this issue of the *Journal,* Dr. David A. Kessler, the commissioner of the Food and Drug Administration, presents his rationale for removing silicone-gel breast implants from the market. Each year about 150,000 women receive these implants—80 percent for the purpose of breast augmentation and almost all the others for reconstruction after mastectomy for cancer. Kessler reminds us that under the 1976 Medical Device Amendments to the federal Food, Drug and Cosmetic Act, manufacturers are required to demonstrate the safety and effectiveness of drugs and devices. Since breast implants were already on the market in 1976, their manufacturers were given extra time to do so. In his view, they have not.

Demonstrating the safety and effectiveness of a drug or device does not, of course, mean showing that there are no side effects or risks. If that were the standard, we would have no drugs or devices, since nearly all of them have possible adverse effects. In evaluation of the balance, risks and benefits are usually considered separately, then weighed.

Kessler argues persuasively that the risks have not been adequately defined, although he points to preliminary findings suggesting that in 4 to 6 percent of asymptomatic women with implants the devices have ruptured. He does not speak to the consequences of rupture or leakage except to say that "the link, if any, between these implants and immune-related disorders and other systemic diseases is...unknown." There is clearly a disparity between the little that has been demonstrated about the risks and the abundance of anecdotes now being related in the media and the courts.

Kessler says even less about the benefits of breast implants. He clearly believes that the benefits are greater for reconstruction after mastectomy than for augmentation, because implants are "an accepted component of cancer therapy." (This is not quite the case, since a mastectomy can be performed, and usually is, without reconstruction.) As Kessler points out, it can be argued that for both indications the benefit is cosmetic.

It is not surprising that the benefits of breast implants get such short shrift. The reason is that they are not subject to analysis in the same way as most treatments for disease. A new treatment can usually be evaluated by a randomized clinical trial, in which objective outcomes are tallied, both risks and benefits. In the case of breast implants, the benefit has to do with personal judgments about the quality of life, which are subjective and unique to each woman. Most women do not wish to have implants, however low the risks, either for augmentation or after mastectomy. Those who do choose to have implants obviously believe there will be substantial benefit, but by its nature this benefit is extremely difficult to assess. The best information we have are polls indicating that more than 90 percent of the women with breast implants are satisfied with the results.

Given the difficulty of assessing the benefits, the FDA has acted as though there were none—at least when implants are used for augmentation. The argument can be made, of course, that the benefit is so small or nebulous that it does not warrant any appreciable risk. But Kessler does not explicitly do that. Instead he implicitly weighs the risks and benefits as though it were so. The result is that he may be holding breast implants to an impossibly high standard: since there are no benefits, there should be no risks.

The fact that any benefits of breast implants are subjective does not mean there are none, as Kessler seems to agree in the case of reconstructive implants. For breast reconstruction, the FDA will permit women to receive implants, but only if they agree to participate in controlled clinical studies. Later, a small number of women who desire implants for augmentation may also have access to a study. All women who receive implants will become part of a registry and will be required to undergo close follow-up.

This approach would be entirely reasonable if breast implants were a new device under evaluation. But that is not the case. They have been on the market for 30 years, and 1 to 2 million women have received them. These facts, as well as the nature of the devices, create several special problems with the FDA's decision.

First, the decision has the effect of coercing women with breast cancer to become subjects of clinical studies, since this is the only way they can receive implants after mastectomy. Yet, according to federal regulations for the protection of human subjects, participation in clinical studies must be entirely voluntary. Although participating in the studies the FDA contemplates will not involve risks any greater than those of receiving implants outside a trial, it will involve the necessity of being available for a follow-up and whatever loss of privacy and inconvenience that entails. To be sure, participation in trials is often the only way for a patient to receive a new drug or device, but this restriction will be perceived differently in the case of breast implants, which are not new.

Second, the FDA's decision has given rise to great fears among the 1 million women now living with implants—fears that in many women are out of all possible proportion to what is known about the risks. The results are hundreds of high-stakes court cases, as well as a lucrative business in removing implants and desperation among those who cannot afford this procedure (the charge may be $5,500). The FDA recommended that women not have their implants removed, but this must seem to many women an anemic reassurance after the dramatic act of withdrawing them from the market. The fact is that the FDA's decision is widely seen as official confirmation that breast implants are dangerous, despite Kessler's assertion that it simply reflects a lack of evidence.

Third, the FDA's decision ignores the social context. Targeting a device used only by women raises the specter of sexism—either in having permitted the use of implants in the first place or in withdrawing them. The view that it is sexist to withdraw implants is exacerbated by the fact that people are regularly permitted to take risks that are probably much greater than the likely risk from breast implants; they do so when they smoke cigarettes, for example, or drink alcohol to excess. The argument that many of these lie outside the purview of the FDA may be seen by many to be a legalism.

David Kessler has been a remarkably effective commissioner, and it is easy to sympathize with the view that he had no choice but to remove breast implants from the market in view of the FDA's finding that their safety and effectiveness have not been demonstrated. And it is also easy to sympathize with irritation that the manufacturers have not been more responsible. But the fact is that Kessler had the discretion to decide either way. The decision was a matter of judgment that he himself acknowledges was "especially difficult."

I believe that the FDA should have permitted women to continue to receive breast implants, regardless of participation in studies and regardless of whether the purpose is augmentation or reconstruction, with the provision that they receive the same information as they would in a trial. And what might that information be? Since we have had more than 30 years of experience with breast implants in more than 1 million women, it is not as though we had no information whatsoever. Women could be told what is known, unsatisfactory though that may be. This would include the estimation of a rate of rupture of 4 to 6 percent and the fact that there are anecdotes about immune disorders caused by a leak or rupture. Perhaps most important, a feeling could be conveyed of an upper bound on the frequency and seriousness of these consequences—based on the paucity of verified cases, as Fisher emphasizes elsewhere in this issue of the *Journal*. Information would also include the finding that women who receive breast augmentation are apparently not at increased risk of cancer, as Berkel et al. report, also in this issue, and the results of the polls showing widespread satisfaction among women with breast implants.

Feminists have been sharply divided on the issue of breast implants. Many applaud the FDA's decision on the grounds that it protects women from taking risks with their health to augment their breasts according to sexist standards. Others object to the decision because they believe it patronizes women. I believe that these views and the underlying concern they represent are not mutually exclusive. It is possible to deplore the pressures that women feel to conform to a stereotyped standard of beauty, while at the same time defending their right to make their own decisions.

SPECIAL REPORT
THE BASIS OF THE FDA'S DECISION ON BREAST IMPLANTS

by David A. Kessler, MD
Commissioner, Food and Drug Administration

On April 16, 1992, the Food and Drug Administration announced that breast implants filled with silicone gel would be available only through controlled clinical studies and that women who need such implants for breast reconstruction would be assured of access to these studies. This decision was especially difficult because even after more than 30 years of use involving more than 1 million women, adequate data to demonstrate the safety and effectiveness of these devices do not exist. They had been allowed to remain on the market after the enactment of the 1976 Medical Device Amendments ("grandfathered") with the understanding that the FDA would later go back and require their manufacturers to submit data demonstrating safety and effectiveness.

Although the decision to limit access to breast implants was in step with the recommendations of an FDA advisory panel, it was one of the most controversial decisions ever made by the agency. It has left the FDA open to criticism on both flanks: from those who argue that the FDA should not let any woman have breast implants as long as their safety and effectiveness

Reprinted with permission from the *New England Journal of Medicine*, June 18, 1992. Copyright 1992, by the Massachusetts Medical Society.

have not been demonstrated, and from those who argue that women ought to be free to weigh the known risks against the personal benefits of an implant and make an independent choice about whether to have one.

The legal basis for the FDA's decision was straightforward. The 1976 Medical Device Amendments to the Food, Drug and Cosmetic Act require that medical devices be shown by their manufacturers to be safe and effective before they may be distributed and used. The legal standard is not that devices must be proved unsafe before the FDA can protect patients against their use. Rather, the law requires a positive demonstration of safety—and the burden of proof rests squarely with the manufacturer. What many participants in this debate have failed to recognize is that under the law, "grandfathered" devices such as breast implants must eventually meet the same requirements as new devices: they must be shown to be safe.

Thirty years after silicone breast implants appeared on the market, the list of unanswered questions about their safety remains long. It is not known how long these devices last, nor is it known what percentage of them will rupture—though it is known that some do rupture. Although manufacturers' reports suggest a frequency of asymptomatic rupture between 0.2 and 1.1 percent, preliminary findings presented at the FDA advisory panel's meeting in February suggested that in 4 to 6 percent of asymptomatic women with implants the devices have ruptured. It is never possible to predict with certainty how a device will function 10, 20, or 30 years after its implantation; however, even basic characteristics that have some value in predicting future performance, such as tensile strength and fatigue resistance tested through cyclic loading, are lacking in this case. The chemical composition of the gel that leaks into the body when a breast implant ruptures is unknown. And the link, if any, between these implants and immune-related disorders and other systemic diseases is also unknown. Serious questions remain about the ability of manufacturers to produce the device reliably and under strict quality controls. Until these questions are answered, the FDA cannot legally approve the general use of breast implants filled with silicone gel.

Nevertheless, to answer these questions once and for all and to preserve the option of access to silicone breast implants for patients whose need is greatest, the FDA has decided to make these devices available under controlled conditions. In the first stage, already in effect, silicone-gel implants will be available to women whose need for them is most urgent. This group includes patients with temporary breast-tissue expanders—whether they were put in place before or during the recent moratorium on the use of silicone breast implants—who are awaiting permanent reconstructive surgery; patients who undergo reconstructive surgery at the time of mastectomy; and those who require the device for urgent medical reasons, as in the case of the rupture of a device already in place. During the second stage, women who desire implants for breast reconstruction will be able to obtain them through extended-availability protocols under the public-health-need provision of the Food, Drug and Cosmetic Act. Under these protocols, silicone-gel implants will be made available to patients with certified medical need for these devices; their registration will be required for the purpose of long-range data collection and follow-up. In the third stage, which includes more intensive research protocols enrolling a limited number of women, the FDA will offer implants for purposes of reconstruction or augmentation in carefully controlled clinical trials. The number of subjects in these studies will be limited to the minimum needed to answer the scientific questions at issue.

Some who criticize the FDA's decision argue that no one should be exposed to a risk that he or she cannot assess. Because we lack information, and because the information we do have arouses concern, the argument claims that women cannot provide valid informed consent when so much information about silicone implants is lacking.

It is true that women who receive implants under the new protocols will be taking a risk of unknown magnitude. It is equally true that, henceforth, any woman entering the clinical trials will be told that implants are not risk-free—a decided improvement over the previous state of "informed consent." The authors of the Medical Device Amendments of 1976 anticipated precisely this type of situation when they included in the law a special exception to the requirements that devices already in use before 1976 had to be demonstrated to be safe and effective in order to remain on the market. The law gives the FDA the prerogative to decide that there is a legitimate public health need for the continued availability of a particular device and, thus, that it may be allowed to remain on the market until studies of its safety and effectiveness are completed.

In allowing patients with cancer and others with a need for breast reconstruction access to silicone breast implants as part of such studies, the FDA has judged that, for these patients, the risk-benefit ratio permits the use of the implant under carefully controlled conditions. In reaching this decision, the FDA carefully weighed whether any alternatives to silicone-gel breast implants existed. Saline implants remain on the market, and for some patients they provide a good alternative to silicone implants. But two additional factors influenced the decision. First, for a small number of patients, silicone implants may be more desirable than saline implants, and second, the safety of saline implants has also not yet been established.

Some argue, however, that it is inconsistent for the FDA to allow the use of a medical device in some situations and not in others. In their view, healthy women who have poor body images because they have small or asymmetrical breasts have as great a need for the device as women who have breast cancer. This contention has a superficial appeal. Although one can legitimately argue for a continuum of need, in the end the needs of the patient who desires reconstructive surgery differ from those of the patient who desires augmentation. One can argue that for both groups the benefit is ultimately cosmetic, yet for women with breast cancer who undergo mastectomy, the option of reconstructive surgery is viewed as an integral part of the treatment of the disease. Certainly, as a society, we are far from according cosmetic interventions the same importance as a matter of public health that we afford to cancer treatments. The clearest demonstration of this social consensus comes from our policies regarding health insurance. In almost any context, the treatment of cancer - and usually reconstruction after mastectomy - is covered as a medical benefit by insurers. But in almost no context is cosmetic surgery, including primary breast augmentation, covered by insurance. It makes little sense for the FDA to consider breast augmentation of equivalent importance with an accepted component of cancer therapy.

These restrictions on the use of silicone-gel implants for breast augmentation are not based on any judgment about values. Rather, the FDA has concluded that women who desire breast augmentation are at higher risk than patients with breast cancer who have had a mastectomy. Unlike patients who have undergone mastectomy, they still have breast tissue, and the presence of an implant complicates the use of mammography for the detection of breast cancer. Although special techniques for more complete mammography have been developed, many experts continue to believe that breast implants can preclude full visualization of the breast. In addition, we are concerned about "silent rupture," the undetected failure of the device in women who have no symptoms of rupture. Mammography is the only reliable procedure for detecting silent rupture, but mammography is not advisable for young women with breast tissue because it entails incremental exposure to radiation. In the end, it comes down to this: in our opinion the risk-benefit ratio does not at this time favor the unrestricted use of silicone breast implants in healthy women.

It has become fashionable in some quarters to argue that women ought to be able to make such decisions on their own. If members of our society were empowered to make their own decisions about the entire range of products for which the FDA has responsibility, however, then the whole rationale for the agency would cease to exist. People could simply communicate directly with manufacturers to design their own drug regimens or select medical devices. The rule governing intervention would be "caveat emptor."

The FDA was established as a result of a social mandate. Caveat emptor has never been—and will never be—the philosophy at the FDA. Manufacturers have vested interests. Between those interests and the interests of patients, the FDA must be the arbiter. To argue that people ought to be able to choose their own risks, that government should not intervene, even in the face of inadequate information, is to impose an unrealistic burden on people when they are most vulnerable to manufacturers' assertions: when they are desperately ill, when they are hoping against hope for a cure, or when they are seeking to enhance their physical appearance. Those are precisely the situations in which the legal and ethical justification for the FDA's existence is greatest, however. The decision about breast implants reflects that need.

Another factor carries equal weight. Had the FDA failed to intervene, the uncontrolled and widespread availability of breast implants would probably have continued for another 30 years— without producing any meaningful clinical data about their safety and effectiveness. Such a situation is obviously unacceptable. Once and for all, we need to gether information about the safety and effectiveness of these medical devices that have been so widely used for so many years.

SILICONE : FRIEND OR FOE?

STRANGE HISTORY OF SILICONE HELD MANY WARNING SIGNS

By Philip J. Hilts

Special to *The New York Times*
January 18, 1992

WASHINGTON, Jan. 17—For decades, doctors and scientists have thought it unlikely anything as inert as silicon could cause significant health problems.

Besides breast implants, silicone plastics made from silicon have been used in valves, tubes and artificial parts in the body. How did the safety of silicone come to be taken for granted if indeed it should not have been?

Looking back at the long medical history of silicone, it is now clear there were many warning signs, some of which were acted on, some of which may have wrongly been overlooked.

In the medical literature of the past 20 years, there has been a rising number of papers on silicon, the element; silicone, the flexible compound built of silicon molecule; and human illness.

Although implant makers maintain that their products are safe, some doctors link silicone in breast implants to a variety of conditions in which the immune system reacts, like arthritis, scleroderma and lupus.

According to company documents, even Dow Corning, the leading implant maker, thought silicone might provoke some kind of immune response. One division of the company tested numerous silicone compounds for use as a booster to vaccines. Such boosters are used to heighten the immune response beyond that of the vaccine itself. The tests did show the compounds had some immune-boosting effect.

[However,] in studies begun in the 1970's Dr. John Paul Heggers of the University of Texas medical campus at Galveston showed that the human immune system reacted to the silicone in breast implants by making antibodies against it. The antibodies attack the silicone and the body's own tissues associated with it.

Starting in 1978, Dr. Heggers said, he wrote and talked to officials of Dow Corning, asking them to take an interest in the possibility that such autoimmune problems resulted from the implants.

"They just weren't interested," he said.

Dr. Robert LeVier, technical chief of the Dow Corning Corporation's Health Care Businesses, said. . . : "That he couldn't get us interested is a pretty accurate statement. We prefer to do our own immunological work here. We disagree with Dr. Heggers on the scientific approach to the problem."

Instead, the company has looked at symptoms that might develop when animals are exposed to silicone. The company's large-scale studies comparing women who have implants and women who do not began only a few months ago, after the recent wave of publicity about implants.

Dr. Heggers said that the meaning of his immune system research is "difficult to say because we don't have a large enough sample of women." He said it is possible that some women are especially prone to immune problems that silicone could trigger, while others could have implants with few ill effects.

"But just because penicillin causes anaphylactic shock sometimes doesn't mean you take penicillin off the market," he said. "We need to identify the sensitive women." At a guess, he said, there may be a few thousand women who have had these problems. . . . It is . . . clear that there are a number of unquestionable hazards of gel-filled silicone breast implants.

A . . . deadly hazard is that silicone is opaque to X-rays, and thus makes mammograms to find early breast cancer very difficult. Dr. Melvin J. Silverstein of the Breast Center in Van Nuys, Calif., who has studied the problem extensively, said that, on average, by the time cancer is discovered in a woman with implants the tumors are five to six times the volume of the tumors found in women without implants. Worse, among patients he studied, 45 percent with implants had cancer that had already spread to the lymph nodes at the time of diagnosis. In women without implants whose cancer was caught by mammography, the cancer had spread only in 6 percent of the cases.

. . . researchers like Dr. Silverstein [still] think women should be able to weigh the risks and choose breast implants if they want them.

The story of silicone began in the 1930's, when scientists at Corning Glass were looking for a caulking material to use as mortar between its fashionable glass blocks. Silicone was considered because it withstood extremes of temperature and retained its properties remarkably well.

Silicones are chains of silicon molecules with side-groups of other molecules. Silicones are versatile; the molecules can be linked up in relatively short chains, which make rather runny liquid, or into much longer chains, which are more rigid and make materials like rubber bands or solid rubber blocks.

Silicone turned out not to be a good substitute for mortar, and silicone in that form remained a laboratory curiosity until the 1950's, when it went on the market as "Silly Putty."

But scientists had taken another look at silicone in World War II when the military asked Corning Glass and Dow Chemical to seek substitutes for scarce rubber. One of the first forms of silicone developed in this effort was a liquid used as an insulator in transformers. At the end of the war, the silicone was used in transformers throughout the nation's electrical network.

The next step in the odyssey detours through the realms of sex and psychology: silicone was used to increase the breast size of Japanese prostitutes. Dr. Edward Kopf, a plastic surgeon in Las Vegas who has made a hobby of the history of silicone, said Japanese cosmetologists realized that American servicemen preferred women with larger breasts than was common among Japanese women. After experimenting with goats' milk, paraffin and a variety of other substances, they tried silicone, injecting it directly into the breast. Soon transformer fluid began disappearing from the Navy's docks in Japan, Dr. Kopf said.

American plastic surgeons began to pick up the Japanese practice, and during the 1960's and 70's, United States literature became littered with grotesque stories and pictures of women with lumpy, ulcerated breasts and scars and other problems in their abdomen, chest, arms and back from the drifting sticky bits of silicone. In a few cases in which the silicone migrated to the lungs, the result was death.

Often, the liquid silicone was mixed with other materials in hope that the resulting inflammation and scar tissue would prevent the formation and migration of lumps.

Doctors working for Dow Corning Corporation contended that problems associated with the injections arose from the other materials, and the company continued to make silicone for injection until it was made illegal, first in Nevada, where many of the worst cases were, then in California, and finally by the Food and Drug Administration.

But researchers continued to seek medical uses for silicone. In 1962, Dr. Frank Gerow and Dr. Thomas Cronin, who later joined Dow Corning, combined rubbery and liquid silicone to create a gel that was soft but firm. They wrapped this gel in a thin envelope of the rubbery silicone polymer, usually referred to as the "elastomer." This was the first silicone gel breast implant. Though the implant has been modified, the basic form is the one that was in use until the F.D.A. effectively banned the sale of silicone gel implants last week.

Many other medical products were developed from silicone, mostly from the elastomer, including tubes and valves, clips that close fallopian tubes in sterilization surgery, penile prostheses, intraocular lenses and tubing for blood oxygenators and dialysis machines.

Overall, these products worked well. But over the years there were disturbing signs that the silicone they contained could cause problems.

One study involved patients on kidney dialysis in which machines purify the patient's blood, which was pumped through silicone tubing. The researchers found that the patients were getting liver disease at an unusually high rate, and some died of it. Autopsies showed their livers had a large number of silicone particles, later shown to have come from the silicone tubing. When the tubes were replaced with another type, the problem stopped.

Similar problems appeared in cardiac bypass surgery, when silicone was used as an antifoam agent in the device that oxygenates patients' blood. It was found that tiny particles of silicone had entered the body and blocked capillaries, causing tissue damage.

Also significant, from the perspective of the current furor, is the incidence of scleroderma, an autoimmune disease critics of implants say is linked to the devices. Scleroderma, in which the growth of fibrous tissues leads to the thickening of the skin, has historically been associated with silica or silicon, the natural element from which silicone is derived. Of 120 men with scleroderma studied in Germany between 1981 and 1988, 93 of them had direct exposure to silica, either as miners, sandblasters, or similar occupations.

During the years when direct silicone gel injection into the body was popular, many recipients reported a wide variety of reactions, including a few rare cases in which silicone inflamed lung tissue and caused suffocation.

In animal studies, it is clear that tissues around implants or injections become permanently inflamed, with the occasional development of benign tumors and other tissue reaction.

These reactions were recorded by Dow Corning scientists studying dogs, but the information was never accurately presented to the Food and Drug Administration, a top agency official said.

In a study of 38 dogs reported in 1973, Dow Corning scientists found that virtually all showed inflammatory reactions. Four dogs were given gel implants; one showed damage to internal organs and died of unknown causes, one formed a benign tumor, and two had inflammation even after two years. But the F.D.A. official said Dow scientists misreported the study, saying that the dogs' health was normal, with only slight inflammation seen.

Rheumatologists and immunologists say it is not clear whether reactions like the benign tumors indicate a full-scale immune reaction. In 1978 Dr. Robert LeVier of Dow acknowledged to the F.D.A. that studies on immune reactions should be carried out to determine what risks women were taking by using implants, but they were not begun until years later.

Those who do not believe silicone can cause true autoimmune disease say there is no doubt that foreign material in the immune system can cause some reaction, but they say the reaction is mostly local and mostly a response of cells like macrophages whose job is to devour foreign materials.

They say full immune system disease is not proven unless there is evidence of antibodies to silicone in large numbers and evidence of lymphocytes, the messengers of full-scale immune response.

More definitive, of course, would be a large-scale study of women with autoimmune diseases, to see whether women with implants were overrepresented. Such studies have been recommended for more than a decade, even by Dow Corning scientists. But the company began such research only a few months ago.

The only big studies of women that the company has carried out were five studies of a total of about 1,000 women. A consultant to Dow Corning called these data the crux of Dow's claims of safety and effectiveness of the implants.

But for the most part, these studies were not of women at all, but instead studies of the records of plastic surgeons. The records were checked to see if women reported any hardness of the breast or other obvious problems. The women themselves were not questioned or examined for the studies, which did not include symptoms of autoimmune diseases.

Dr. Steven Weiner, chief of rheumatology at the School of Medicine at the University of California at Los Angeles, said that he has treated about 60 women with implants who have scleroderma or other autoimmune disorders. Although it is far from proven that the implants caused their disease, he said, half to two-thirds of the women showed much improvement after the implants were removed. Dr. Nir Kossovsky, a specialist in biomaterials and pathology at U.C.L.A., said it was possible that it was not the silica or silicone itself that was causing problems. It may be that, once in the body, these materials attract proteins from the body itself which then become wrapped around the silicone. It is these proteins to which the body may mount an autoimmune reaction, and the reaction may spill over to the rest of the body. That is, the immune cells attack the proteins in other parts of the body as well.

Dr. Noel R. Rose, professor and chairman of the Department of Immunology at Johns Hopkins School of Hygiene and Public Health, and who has testified in court on behalf of Dow Corning, said Dr. Kossovsky may be correct but it would be difficult to prove it.

"Should the company have done more, earlier?" he asked. "Should the F.D.A have pushed them harder to get the data? I just don't have a good feel for why we are left 20 years on, still saying we are sorry, we wish these things would have been looked at 20 years ago."

SILICONE
A SIMPLIFIED LOOK AT
A MODERN MATERIAL

Dr. Kenneth R. Carter

IBM Research Division,
Almaden Research Center
1992

Recently there has been a great deal of controversy surrounding the use of breast implant devices which incorporate silicone. While most people have heard the basic arguments on the pros and cons of such implants, few actually know what silicone is.

Silicones are a group of materials belonging to a class of substances known as polysiloxanes. Polysiloxanes are polymers, materials that consist of long chains of connected atoms. Commonly, polymers are referred to as plastics, rubbers, oils or glues.

Polymers consist of very long chains of carbon, nitrogen and oxygen atoms; these polymers include polystyrene, nylon or vinyl polymers. Each polymer has different properties that depend upon what order the atoms are linked to one another as well the length of the chains . . . As a rule, the longer the chain of atoms is, the stronger and less flexible the polymer will be.

Silicones, better referred to as polysiloxanes, are polymers that consist of links of the atoms silicon (si) and oxygen.

Though polysiloxanes have carbon atoms present, it is the linked silicon and oxygen atoms that set these polymers apart from other types of polymers.

The atom silicon makes up over a quarter of the earth's crust and is the basic component of sand and glass. Polysiloxanes, however, are not naturally occurring materials but they have been in commercial production since the 1940's.

Polysiloxanes are of great importance due to the unique properties these materials possess, which in turn are due to the silicon-oxygen linkages. Depending upon the exact chemical structure and chain lengths, polysiloxanes can be tailor-made to oils, greases, or solid rubbers. Among the many unique properties of polysiloxanes are stability to high temperatures, water repellency, and chemical inertness. Therefore, common uses include car polishes, water-proofing coatings, window sealants, caulking compounds, non-stick cooking sprays and adhesives.

Chemical inertness means that these materials do not react with other chemicals easily. [As a consequence,] they have always been considered non-toxic and have been used in many biomedical applications in which the use of many other common polymers is impractical. Though one of its best known biomedical applications is in breast implant devices, the use of silicone rubbers in parts for artificial hearts and other medical organs is extremely important because polysiloxanes are more stable in living systems than other polymers.

Polysiloxanes or silicones are a very important class of materials which fulfill needs that other materials cannot. . . . it is important to know that silicones have many uses and properties. . . . their use has greatly benefited society, and will continue to do so.

BIOMEDICAL APPLICATIONS OF SYNTHETIC POLYMERS

by Harry R. Allcock and
Frederick W. Lampe

from *Contemporary Polymer Chemistry*, 1981

The widespread use of synthetic polymers in technology and in everyday life is an accepted feature of modern civilization. Polymers are now being used for almost every conceivable application, and there is every indication that these uses will continue to increase in future years. However, there exists one important area in which the use of synthetic polymers has generally been cautious and limited—the area of medicine. There are a number of scientific reasons for this. . . . The important point is that profound changes are expected in medical techniques as new synthetic polymers are developed. In fact, the application of polymers to medicine has become one of the principal challenges facing the polymer scientist.

. . . a polymer must fulfill certain critical requirements if it is to be used in an artificial organ.

First, it must be physiologically inert. Nearly all synthetic polymers suffer from one common disadvantage—their ability to trigger off rejection mechanisms by the body. These rejection processes become manifest in the coagulation of blood in contact with polymers or the inflammation or even tumor formation which occurs when some polymers remain in contact with internal tissues for long periods of time. The overcoming of these deleterious interactions is one of the most urgent problems faced by the synthetic polymer chemist...

Second, the polymer itself should be stable during many years of exposure to hydrolytic or oxidative conditions at body temperature. It must be resistant to enzyme attack, and it must not change dimensions, disintegrate, or dissolve in aqueous media or in contact with lipids or other fatty materials.

It is important to recognize that the use of synthetic polymers in living systems revolves around one of two requirements: that the polymer should be totally inert, or that the polymer should be totally biodegradable. Unfortunately, most polymers fall between these two extremes.

The body has three basic responses to the implantation of a foreign body. First, it responds to the physical characteristics of the object (shape, roughness, presence of sharp edges, etc.). These responses may take the form of epithelial encapsulation of the foreign body, keratinization of the surrounding tissue, thickening of the connective tissue, or generation of giant cells. Second, the body reacts to the chemical toxicity (if any) of the polymer by the appearance of tissue inflammation, inhibition of epithelial growth, and other effects. Finally, there is a possibility of the direct generation of an antigenic reaction by some chemical component of the polymer surface.

Thus, the comparison of different polymers for biomedical uses is not a straight-forward process. Research workers disagree about the relative significance of implant design and the chemical properties of the material. They also disagree on the question of whether demonstrated tumor formation in rodents means that some polymers will initiate tumor growth in human beings. Human metabolism is much slower than that of rodents, although human beings live much longer. Add to this the complication

that many commercial polymers contain potentially toxic or
carcinogenic monomers or additives that can be leached out
easily in the body, and it will be seen that enormous difficulties
face the researcher who wishes to answer the question: Which
polymer is the best for a particular biomedical application?

With these uncertainties it will be recognized that the
following observations are tentative indeed. Tissue culture experiments suggest that the following order represents an *increasing* degree of toxicity of various polymers:

> *Silicone rubber*, polyethylene,
> poly(tetrafluoroethylene)
> fluorinated poly(ethylene-propylene)
> poly(phenylene oxide)
> poly(methyl methacrylate) < poly(vinylidene fluoride)
> nylon, polystyrene, *polyurethane*
> poly(vinyl chloride)
> ABS polymer.

Those toward the end of the list totally inhibited the growth
of tissue culture cells.

Of course, the interaction between a polymer and the body
may also lead to a weakening of the polymer itself. Polyurethanes disintegrate after only 16 months in the body. . . .
Silicone rubber, on the other hand, is hardly affected at all in a
year and a half in the body.

MAMMARY IMPLANTS

By Nir Kossovsky and Nora Papasian

Mammary implants in the 1990s are highly controversial medical devices. The public debate has deteriorated to calls for freedom of choice, demands for definitive evidence of harm by proponents, and charges of corporate malfeasance by critics. Underlying this spectacle, however, is a 30-year treasure of biophysical experiments, animal trials, and clinical human experience. What matters most is that the reader understands that (a) neither silicone nor polyester polyurethanes are inert materials; (b) the full clinical spectrum of silicone and polyurethane associated phenomena have not yet been defined; (c) materials other than silicone may have superior mechanical and bioreactivity properties; and (d) that in view of the current silicone crisis, concerted biological testing of existing and new materials would seem advisable.

Inflammation is the expected biological reaction to an implanted mammary prosthesis. Although acute inflammation is the initial response to any implantation because of the associated surgical trauma, the chronic phase is the significant biological response to mammary implants that are intended for long-term

Reprinted by permission of *Journal of Applied Biomaterials*, Vol. 3, xxx-xxx (1992), John Wiley & Sons, Inc., New York.

or even lifetime use. The primary cells mediating the chronic inflammatory response are the macrophage and lymphocyte. The macrophage is especially important. As an avid scavenger, the macrophage attempts to engulf the implant or components thereof, such as polyurethane foam fragments, silicone bleed, or free gel. But when the components of the implant are much larger than the macrophage and not easily [engulfed], as is the case with the silicone rubber surface of breast implants, fibrous scar tissue encapsulates and isolates the material. As this tissue capsule contracts as part of the wound-healing process, it begins to attain the shape of minimal surface area as dictated by physical principles: a sphere. In approximately 40% of the implanted patients, the contracture is significant enough to force the pliable breast implant to conform, yielding varying degrees of roundness and an unnatural appearing breast mass . . . [This] is termed *capsular contracture.*

. . . gel bleed can not be prevented. Bleeding is a natural phenomenon—the diffusion of small molecules through a semipermeable membrane. . . . The smaller/short low molecular weight chains [of polymers] . . . diffuse through the rubber shell.

. . . The macrophages may engulf the silicone and remain quiescent; . . . or they may process the engulfed silicone [and] elicit an immunological response. . . . [Less] than favorable outcomes . . . have been widely reported anecdotally. The reactions vary from erythema to lumps to interstitial pneumonitis.

Silicones tend to spread once introduced into the biological environment. They may spread locally through soft tissues, may migrate to lymph nodes, or may enter the vascular system through various routes. Oils and gels . . . will travel more easily through tissue planes and the vasculature. Thus, in addition to intensifying the local reactions elicited by the rubber, silicone gel threatens to cause systemic reactions.

Systemic reactions . . . may be due to biological sensitization to the emulsified silicone-protein complexes. In this scenario, proteins denatured upon binding to the surface of silicone gel droplets are [engulfed] by macrophages, who then present the complex as antigen to immune competent lymphocytes. The consequence of this process may be any one of the four types of hypersensitivity reactions including autoimmunity, although experimental evidence for antibody production and type IV delayed hypersensitivity) only have been accumulated to date.

The known fragmentation and progressive degradation of the polyester polyurethane used for implant fabrication may explain the material's seeming success in delaying capsule formation and contracture, but they have also stirred a myriad of questions regarding possible complications. . . . FDA studies suggest that the foam degrades to toluene diamine spontaneously, and some individuals have reported detecting toluene diamine in both the urine and breast milk of implant bearers. Peak TDA urine concentrations have been reported to occur during the first few weeks following implantation and have been attributed to unpolymerized monomers leaching from the newly implanted device. Others, in particular the manufacturer, have argued that the TDA being measured in the urine is an artifact of the analytic process. . . . For those concerned about the health effects of TDA, this position should not afford excessive comfort. . . . Overall, the value of urine or breast milk TDA analysis is not clear at present [although] TDA is a potent animal carcinogen . . .

Owing to a popular misconception that silicone is an inert material, research into the development of superior materials for implantable breast prostheses has been inhibited. From the current vantage point, it appears that materials other than silicone may have superior mechanical and bioreactivity properties. Investigators should feel challenged to identify, develop, and validate the safety of these new materials.

PLASTIC SURGEONS HAD WARNINGS ON SAFETY OF SILICONE IMPLANTS

By Joan E. Rigdon

Staff Reporter of
The Wall Street Journal
March 12, 1992

While the silicone-implant debate has focused on whether manufacturers hid suspected risks from the public, there is evidence that over the past two decades, plastic surgeons themselves saw and ignored red flags in this lucrative branch of their specialty. Critics say many plastic surgeons failed to alert women to possible health risks reported by several sources, including professional journals, manufacturers and some of their own patients.

Some evidently continue to do so. This newspaper sent a reporter to four randomly chosen plastic-surgery offices in New York City, presenting herself as a candidate for implant surgery. The surgeons didn't recommend silicone-gel implants, on which the FDA has imposed a moratorium. But all four recommended saline implants, which are essentially silicone bags filled with saline solution. None mentioned Food and Drug Administration warnings that saline implants with silicone exteriors may interfere with mammograms and may pose an increased risk of cancer and autoimmune disorders.

Critics say that the American Society of Plastic and Recon

structive Surgeons has emphasized promotion of breast implants over investigation of their safety. The ASPRS is collecting millions of dollars from its members to lobby to keep the devices on the market.

"The ASPRS operated like a commercial enterprise rather than a collegial medical society," says Jane Sprague Zones, a medical sociologist at the University of California at San Francisco and a board member of the National Women's Health Network. Ms. Zones served as the consumer representative on the FDA advisory panel that recently recommended restricting use of silicone implants to breast cancer patients and medical experiments.

Doctors are quick to point out that they couldn't inform patients of risks they didn't know about, such as Dow Corning Corp. researchers' previously secret fears that implants could leak or burst, sending silicone through the body with unknown consequences.

But Dow Corning wasn't the only entity studying implants. Dozens of case studies published in medical journals over the past two decades describe a litany of problems that may be associated with silicone-gel implants, including skin rashes, swollen breasts, hardened breasts, severe joint pain, chronic fatigue and debilitating immune disorders. Even manufacturers' product literature warned of some possible ill effects of silicone implants, but many patients say these warnings were never passed along to them.

Plastic surgeons point out that it still isn't known what health risks, if any, are associated with silicone gel implants. They say that if reports of risks were downplayed, that's because the reports weren't scientifically documented. And if they neglected to tell patients of risks outlined in product literature, that's because "there's a feeling a lot of things in [product literature] may overly alarm patients," says Norman Cole, president of the ASPRS.

Silicone-gel breast-implant surgery can bring a surgeon anywhere from $1,000 to $7,500 for a few hours' work. Some plastic surgeons say privately that this was a powerful temptation to dismiss anecdotal reports of problems.

Anecdotal evidence of trouble surfaced regularly in the medical literature. In 1979, for instance, the *Annals of Plastic Surgery* published a report by Barry Uretsky, a Pittsburgh cardiologist, describing how one patient suffered fevers, sweats, swollen joints and enlarged kidneys within days of getting silicone-gel implants. She almost died, the report said, but recovered seven weeks after her implants were removed. In 1986, the *Journal of Plastic and Reconstructive Surgery* published a paper by Steven R. Weiner, a rheumatologist at the University of California, Los Angeles, documenting cases of three silicone-implant patients who had joint pain, including one who lost partial use of an arm.

That same year Dr. Silverstein, an oncologist at the Breast Center in Van Nuys, Calif., presented his group's findings that implants can interfere with mammograms to a meeting of plastic surgeons in Los Angeles. Dr. Silverstein recalls: "They said, 'That's ridiculous. Go back to the laboratory and study it again. You're going to chase all the patients out of our offices.'" He did go back to the laboratory, and has repeatedly come to the same conclusion, which is now gaining acceptance among plastic surgeons.

Mr. Rudy, the former president of Heyer-Schulte Corp., says he became alarmed about the safety of his own company's silicone implants after surgeons returned 140 ruptured implants, asking for replacements, in a 13-month period ending June 1976. In August 1976, he wrote the surgeons a letter asking for more information on how the implants had broken and how long they were implanted before breaking. The letter warned that "currently available mammary prostheses are not perfect" and that "doctors and patients should expect that some patients will exhibit some adverse response to silicone implants." Attached was a bibliography of medical journal articles.

But his customers didn't want to make safety an issue, Mr. Rudy contends. "Plastic surgeons were willing to discuss problems by pulling you aside and saying 'between us girls,' " he says. "But they didn't want to openly criticize. They felt any problem that occurred might hurt their own business."

Undoubtedly, many women have researched silicone implants, calculated the risk-to-reward ratio and decided to go ahead with the surgery. For others the desire for larger breasts may outweigh the risks. "I definitely let people know about very real complications, but they tend to be so single-minded of purpose that they sort of hear it with one ear," says Robert S. Hoffman, a psychiatrist at the Breast Center. Recently, he says, he tried to discourage a physically fit 22-year-old who worked out constantly and wanted breast implants because her mother made fun of her bra size. "I felt there were a lot of things to work on" psychologically, Dr. Hoffman says. "But she rationalized [the need for surgery] 700 ways."

Many women agree that they sought implants to improve their figures and self-esteem, but wish they had been told of the risks before lying down on the operating table. Lisa VanSyoc, a Phoenix entrepreneur who got silicone implants covered with polyurethane in 1990, says she got them because she "hated looking at that 12-year-old body on a 28-year-old women."

At the office of Phoenix plastic surgeon James E. Cessna, Ms. VanSyoc says, she was shown a video featuring women talking about how bigger breasts had improved their self-esteem. Then, she says, a doctor's aide gave her a short speech on the surgery, dismissed worries that implants might be associated with rheumatoid arthritis and quickly flipped through a binder of pictures of women with implants. "I felt like I was on a conveyor belt," Ms. VanSyoc says.

Dr. Cessna declines to discuss her case, citing doctor-patient confidentiality, but says he and his staff spend two hours with each patient informing her of the risks such as implant rupture, silicone spreading, loss of nipple sensation and dependency on steroids, which are used to treat inflamed breasts.

Ms. VanSyoc chose another Phoenix doctor, John A. Ward,

who inserted polyurethane-coated silicone implants. She says Dr. Ward performed the operation without reviewing product literature listing risks, including infections, muscle pain, swelling, "neural changes," possible dislodging of the implant, rupture and silicone leakage with "unknown" long-term health effects.

The surgical consent form Ms. VanSyoc signed mentioned "a possibility of implant breakage or leakage requiring implant removal or replacement" and stated that "rarely, silicone migration to adjacent tissue occurs." It didn't mention the possibility that her implants might dislodge, which they later did.

Ms. VanSyoc also says her doctor downplayed risks that she might temporarily or permanently lose feeling in parts of her breasts. "Now you could poke me with a knife and I'd stand there and stare at you," she says. Dr. Ward declines to comment, citing doctor-patient confidentiality.

Some women say doctors brushed them aside when they raised questions about implants. Sonia Woodall, a Lexington, Ky., real-estate developer whose implants ruptured, says she went back to the doctor who put them in and complained of symptoms including chronic fatigue, joint pain and the loss of her monthly period. The surgeon, Dr. John Bostwick III of Emory University School of Medicine in Atlanta, "told me I was menopausal and that I should go home and quit reading" about suspected complications of silicone, she says.

Ms. Woodall's husband, Jerry, was in the room at the time and confirms his wife's recollection. Mr. Woodall says that at the time, he agreed with the doctor. Ms. Woodall says she was so angry she left the room without speaking to either the doctor or her husband, and she adds that her period resumed six weeks after she had her implants removed by another doctor. Dr. Bostwick declines to comment, citing doctor-patient confidentiality.

With silicone-implant safety now a hotly debated issue, the American Society of Plastic and Reconstructive Surgeons is sticking to its guns. Dr. Cole, its president, says, "There are no long-term proven ill effects from implants that we know of."

The society has imposed a special levy on its members to raise a war chest of $3.9 million over the next three years; so far, it plans to spend about one-eighth of that on research and the rest on lobbying.

This response has enraged some plastic surgeons, who fear that responding to health concerns with an expensive lobbying campaign demeans the profession. "The energy that went into raising money was absolutely ridiculous," says one ASPRS member, who declines to be named. "I don't believe in fighting. I believe in getting data. Let's get some data for these poor souls."

Says Dr. Cole, "We felt that we had not had any platform before. It seemed like it was time for plastic surgeons and patients to tell the other side."

Aggressive lobbying is nothing new for the ASPRS. In a 1982 petition to the FDA, the late H. William Potterfield, then president of the Society, defined a disease to fit his colleagues' cure. Referring to "the female breast that does not achieve normal or adequate development," he wrote that "there is a substantial and enlarging body of medical information and opinion . . . to the effect that these deformities are really a disease which in most patients result in feelings of inadequacy, lack of self-confidence, distortion of body image and a total lack of well being due to a lack of self-perceived femininity." The ASPRS repudiates that view today.

SOURCE READINGS IN THE HISTORY OF COSMETIC SURGERY

Cosmetic and plastic surgery have been around for a very long time. The desire to improve on Nature, correct deformities, or reconstruct an injury is deeply rooted in the human psyche, both for the victim and the surgeon. The myth of the sculptor Pygmalion, who created his idea of the perfect woman out of nature's raw material, has fascinated and tantalized for centuries. The following excerpts from historical writings describe procedures which continue to be common today—although surgical techniques have certainly improved.

ANCIENT RHINOPLASTIC OPERATIONS IN INDIA

from the *Sushruta Samhitá*
translated by Kaviraj Kunjalal Bhishagratna

Now I shall deal with the process of affixing an artificial nose. First the leaf of a creeper, long and broad enough to fully cover the whole of the severed or clipped off part, should be gathered, and a patch of living flesh, equal in dimension to the preceding leaf should be sliced off (from down upward) from the region of the cheek and, after scarifying it with a knife, swiftly adhered to the severed nose. Then the cool headed physician should steadily tie it up with a bandage decent to look at and perfectly suited to the end for which it has been employed. . . .

The physician should make sure that the adhesion of the severed parts has been fully effected and then insert two small pipes into the nostrils to facilitate respiration, and to prevent the adhesioned flesh from hanging down. After that, the adhesioned part should be dusted with the powders of Pattanga [sappan root], Yashtimadhukam [licorice root], and Rasanjana [barberry] pulverised together, and the nose should be enveloped in Karpasa cotton and several times sprinkled over with the refined oil of pure sesamum. Clarified butter should be given to the patient for drink, and he should be anointed with oil and treated with purgatives after the complete digestion of the meals he has taken . . . Adhesion should be deemed complete after the incidental ulcer has been perfectly healed up, while the nose should be again scarified and bandaged in the case of a semi or partial adhesion. The adhesioned nose should be tried to be elongated where it would fall short of its natural size in the case of the abnormal growth of its newly formed flesh . . .

[Editor's note: The *Sushruta Samhitá* is a three-volume, comprehensive encyclopedia of medicine, believed to have been written in India more than 2,000 years ago, and considered part of the *Vedas*—KO]

THE HISTORY OF BLEPHAROPLASTY TO CORRECT BLEPHAROCHALASIS
EYELID SURGERY BY ARABIC SURGEONS, 10TH AND 11TH CENTURIES AD

By Kathryn L. Stephenson, M.D.
Santa Barbara, California

Surgical relief of the full overhanging eyelid and of puffiness and wrinkling of the lower eye-lid was undertaken by Arabic surgeons of the tenth and eleventh centuries A.D. . . .

Abul Qasim (936-1013), or Albucasis as he is more commonly known, was born in the Andalusian town of Zahra near Cordova [Spain] and was the author of a great medical-surgical treatise called the Al-Tas'rif. . . . In Volume II, Chapter 15, entitled "Cauterization for the Relaxation of the Eyelids," Albucasis wrote as follows:

> In the relaxation of the eyelids following illness or caused by fluid, it is necessary to cauterize a little above the eyelids, two times on each side avoiding approaching the temples. The length of the cauterization will be the length of the eyelids.

. . . Ophthalmology and optics were particularly advanced by the Arabic surgeons, of which Ali ibn-Isa [Baghdad, ca. 940 - 1010 A.D.] was perhaps the most outstanding.

Ali ibn-Isa wrote of blepharoptosis, extraction of cataracts, corneal tattooing to facilitate the sale of slaves, excision of epidermoid cysts, and lagophthalmus. In the 31st chapter entitled "Relaxation (Ptosis) of the Upper Lid (Istirha)," he wrote the following:

> Blepharoptosis of the upper lid results from a relaxation (paralysis) so that it can no longer be raised. Often this enfeeblement is so marked that the lashes turn in and scratch the eyeball. . . .

His reference to the surgery described in Chapter X under trichiasis and its treatment is as follows:

> Having put the patient to sleep, the lid must be everted so that the eyelashes can be firmly grasped between thumb and fingers on the left hand, which at the same time holds a spatula that presses out the middle of the eyelid. Then the lid margin must be split along its whole length with a small knife. If the incision is not made properly and there are irregularities at the ends the central split will fail of its purpose. The next step is to carry out the folding . . . of the lid tissue to be excised. Having determined the position and amount of these, conditioned largely upon the situation and number of false lashes, the latter are to be excised, cutting out most tissue where exuberant hairs are most numerous.
>
> The procedure should be carried out on the upper lid only, and the excision of the parts that lie beneath the introduced threads must be done with scissors.
>
> Moreover it is wise . . . that the awakened patient should be asked to open and close both eyes before the chief or final excisions are made. The lips of the wound are now brought together with three equidistant stitches, the middle one to be tied first. The parts are now covered with yellow powder and a small bandage applied. . . .

THE DEFORMITY TERMED "PUG NOSE" AND ITS CORRECTION, BY A SIMPLE OPERATION

John O. Roe

Medical Record

June 4, 1887

The nose is the central and most prominent feature of the face; and on its shape, size, and appearance, to a great degree, depends the relative facial beauty of the person.

Physiognomists emphasize the importance of the nose in the category of anatomical conformations that are indicative of special traits of character; and regard it as a measure of force in nations and individuals.

Says Wells: "A skillful dissembler may disguise, in a degree, the expression of the mouth; the hat may be slouched over the eyes; the chin may be hidden in a impenetrable thicket of beard; but the nose will stand out 'and make its sign' in spite of all precautions. It utterly refuses to be ignored, and we are, as it were, compelled to give it our attention."

Even in ancient times much attention was given to its shape and appearance. Among the ancient Persians no man who had a crooked or deformed nose was allowed to sit upon the throne. Cyrus, it is said, had an asymmetrical nose, which was made a thing of beauty through the kind assistance of his emasculated attendants. In order to secure symmetrical and handsomely formed noses, in the children of the royal blood, the eunuchs who had charge of the royal offspring were accustomed to mould their noses into perfect shape.

Considered from the profile point of view alone, noses are classified according to their shape by students of physiognomy into five main classes:

1) The Roman noses;
2) The Greek noses;
3 The Jewish noses;
4) The Snub or Pug noses; and
5) The Celestial noses.

These classes of noses, considered in the light of the characteristics of the race or class to which they are peculiar, are observed to indicate prominent traits of character, as follows:

The Roman indicates executiveness or strength; the Greek, refinement; the Jewish, commercialism or desire for gain; the Snub or Pug, weakness and lack of development; the Celestial, weakness, lack of development, and inquisitiveness. . . .

Mr. Warwick says: "A snub-nose is to us a subject of most melancholy interest. We behold in it a proof of a degeneracy of the human race."

Tristram Shandy's father, regretting his son's misfortunes, remarked: "No family, however high, could stand against a succession of short noses;" and his grandfather "when tendering his best hand and heart to the lady who afterward consented to 'make him the happiest of men' was forced to capitulate to her terms owing to the brevity of his nose. . . . "

During development the nose and parts comprising the central portion of the face . . . are late in developing, and are also the last portions of the face to undergo ossification. At birth the nose, at its base and central portions, is flat and nearly level with the face, but later this depressed line is replaced by a more prominent one as the nose becomes developed. From this it will be seen that anything interfering with the upper development of these parts so as to cause them to remain in their infantile condition, while the end of the nose undergoes due development, will give the nose a snubbed and unsightly shape.

The best developed and most beautiful noses are one-third the length of the face. But noses often vary from this proportion, and in some instances an ill-formed nose is inherited, it being a special family mark. . . .

The operation for the correction of the deformity under consideration is easily performed, although I can find no record of it, and have no knowledge of its having been proposed or performed.

It . . . is mainly to improve the personal appearance of the individual.

The operation consists in the removal from the end of the nose that tissue which is in excess, or which is disproportionate in amount to the other portions of the nose. In other words, we are to make the nose symmetrical from one end to the other. . . .

The nose does not appear ugly by reason of the fact that its size is disproportionate to that of the face (for noses vary greatly in this respect), but by reason of the disproportionate relations to one another of the different parts of the nose itself. . . .

The operation is performed as follows: We first deaden the sensibility of the interior of the end of the nose by cocaine (general anaesthesia being unnecessary) and then brightly illuminate this part.

The end of the nose is turned upward and backward, and held with a retractor by an assistant; then sufficient of the superfluous tissue is removed or dissected out to allow the nose to conform to the shape that we desire. Great care must, however, be exercised not to remove too much tissue, and also not to cut through into the skin, lest we may have afterward a scar or a dent in the external surface of the nose.

THE CORRECTION OF ANGULAR DEFORMITIES OF THE NOSE BY A SUBCUTANEOUS OPERATION

John O. Roe

Medical Record

July 18, 1891

It is my purpose to describe to you, in this short paper, an operation for the correction of angular deformities of the nose by a subcutaneous operation.

In describing the technique of this operation, I cannot make it more clear than by briefly reporting some cases in which I have performed the operation. Miss C_____, aged twenty-five, consulted me for a "winter cough," which was giving her much concern. While she was under treatment she often referred to her nose, and complained about an angular, bony projection on its top that not only gave her nose an unsightly shape, but so pierced the skin as to make it painful for her to wash or wipe her face. She was quite desirous of getting rid of the annoying projection, but was afraid an operation might leave an unsightly scar. In order to avoid this possibility, I suggested that the projection be removed by an incision from the inside of the nostril without wounding the skin, and this suggestion at once induced her to have the operation performed.

After anaesthetizing the part with cocaine, both by applying it to the interior of the nostril and by injecting some under the skin with a hypodermic syringe, I made a lineal incision completely through the upper wall of the left nostril, just in front of the nasal bone, between it and the upper lateral cartilage of the nostril, to the under side of the skin. This incision I widened laterally from the insertion of the upper border of the triangular cartilage half-way down the side of the nose, until I had a sufficiently large opening to permit the introduction of instruments freely. I then raised the skin from the bridge of the nose over the region where the operation was to be performed. After the skin was sufficiently freed from the top of the nose I inserted a pair of angular bone scissors and cut off the projecting piece of bone until the top of the nose was perfectly straight and smooth. The operation was done with the strictest antiseptic precautions, and after completion I blew in some iodoform powder, through the opening, over every portion of the wounded surface. The skin was then allowed to drop back upon the bridge of the nose, and, by strapping it down with gentle pressure, the wound healed without the slightest formation of pus, and there was very little soreness. There was no mutilation of the interior of the nose, for even directly after the operation it was difficult to detect, by simply inspecting the interior of the nose, the incision that had been made. In a few days the nose was entirely healed, and the soreness had disappeared when the patient left for her home.

About six weeks afterward she wrote me that she was highly delighted with the result. She no longer had to be constantly on her guard lest she should allow something to come against her nose, and she said that it felt as if she could beat it against a stone wall without hurting it.

FACIAL PLASTIC
SURGERY AND BEAUTY
AN EVOLUTION

	1950'S and 1960's	1970's	Today
EYEBROW/ EYELID SURGERY	• high lidded eyes • lots of space between eye and brow • wide-eyed look • incision line at corner of eye covered by "doe-eye" make-up • incision line visible • eyebrows raised very high	• lid width narrows, brow still slightly high • entire eyelid sculpted rather than lifted for more natural look	• narrower lid • 5 to 6 millimeters of space between brow for eye • natural appearance • incision line extends from upper lid, instead of corner of eye
FACELIFT	• surface changes only • pulled-back, stretched appearance • incision line visible	• uderlying musculature tightened • incisions reconsidered for less obvious scarring • neckline scars still visible	• very natural, non-surgical look • complete scar camouflaging • adjustments more sophisticated
FACIAL SCULPTING	• did not exist	• did not exist	• bone reshaped to improve facelift results • solves facial balance problems not addressed before
NOSE SURGERY	• turned up, ski-jump angle, nostrils showing • cute, childlike • highly sculpted tip	• transition from stylized, uniform result to more aggressive nose	• longer, stronger nose • 90% upward angle • wider bridge • fuller, gently refined tip • individualized nose based on each face • natural, non-surgical look

Courtesy of the American Academy of Facial Plastic and Reconstructive Surgery.

COMMON
PROCEDURES

The following section explains the most commonly sought procedures. Most can be performed on an outpatient basis, although you and your doctor will decide together whether a hospital stay might be better for you. Anesthesia can be either general or local, depending on the extent of the surgery as well as your comfort level. If you are using an outpatient facility, make sure that the doctor has an anesthesiologist or licensed nurse-anesthetist on staff.

ANESTHESIA

One under-emphasized aspect of surgery is anesthesia. Yet this is the most deadly area. A surgeon can make a mistake; he or she can cut in the wrong place, or too much, or not enough; rarely are deaths directly related to the surgeon's technique. A mistake in sedation or anesthesia is much more likely to be fatal.

The purpose of sedation and anesthesia is twofold. Patients want to avoid feeling the pain of the surgery. For the squeamish, a general anesthetic, or going completely to sleep—"wake me up when it's over"—is far preferable to a local which leaves one having to listen to everything that is going on. On the other hand, going completely under is harder on the body in terms of recovery and after-effects. But any level of anesthesia should prevent the patient from consciously feeling the pain.

Surgeons, meanwhile, need a patient to be completely still so that they can work. This can always be achieved with a general anesthetic, taking the patient to a deep level of unconsciousness. However, under sedation and light levels of anesthesia, a patient still has his or her reflex mechanisms and can react to stimuli such as the knife slicing off part of the body. An "excitability" period, one of the lightest levels of anesthesia, doesn't inhibit involuntary responses in which the patient seems to be fighting the doctor, the nurses, and anyone else who attempts restraint. Skip Verne, a nurse-anesthetist based in Beverly Hills, prefers to put his patients under general anesthesia for most procedures. It's just more practical and effective.

An anesthesiologist or nurse-anesthetist should really stay in the office to make sure the patient wakes up after the procedure. Unfortunately, many do not. The odds are that a patient will wake up with no problem, so many anesthesiologists will overbook their time, especially when they work in association with a hospital where there are many other trained personnel to deal with an emergency. In an outpatient setting, this practice can be risky.

Usually, neither the staff nor the surgeon are trained to spot emergency situations relating to the anesthetic, and they are often too busy to check on patients as they are coming out of anesthesia. Recently a breast augmentation patient, whose husband had come to pick her up, was found dead in the recovery room of her doctor's office. She was stiff from rigor mortis when he came to get her.

A good question to ask a potential surgeon, therefore, is how long his or her anesthesiologist stays after a procedure. See if the surgeon uses the same anesthetist for most of his or her procedures. An anesthetist who is virtually "on staff" is a good bet. If you can talk to the anesthesiologist or nurse-anesthetist, ask him or her personally about his/her work habits in this regard. The answer should either comfort you or make you think twice.

A conservative anesthetist will make sure you are talking and even walking on your own before he or she leaves. Tragedies from anesthesia are usually avoidable, and always the result of human error. A closely monitored patient can be resuscitated by re-starting the heart or breathing, or pulled out of an allergic reaction with medication, but the anesthesiologist can't be out to lunch or off to the next case if he expects to keep an eye on what's going on with you.

Your doctor will work with either an MD Anesthesiologist or a nurse-anesthetist. Both are equally qualified to perform your anesthesia. A nurse-anesthetist will be less expensive and more likely to be at least semi-attached to your doctor's office.

Anesthesia is a form of controlled poisoning, says Skip Verne. The anesthesiologist should be allowed all the time he or she needs to ensure that the patient is appropriately sedated. Sometimes patients experience nausea and vomiting after anesthesia, especially with use of drugs from the narcotic family such as morphine or Demerol. Nausea can be prevented or lessened by careful administration of the amount of the drug and also by giving other, anti-emetic drugs both during and immediately following the surgery. If you find yourself suffering excessive nausea or vomiting following a surgery, call your doctor for an anti-emetic. Nausea and vomiting are almost unavoidable after nasal surgery, but not so much from the anesthesia as from the draining of blood down the back of the throat.

Anesthesia can take several forms. You may be sedated with an injection first to relax you or your doctor may have prescribed Valium to take orally before you come to the office. If you are not particularly nervous, these precautions are redundant. Before surgery, an intravenous catheter is inserted in your arm to allow the anesthetic to drip directly into your bloodstream. The anesthesia may be maintained with inhalation, in which a mask is placed over your face and you will be breathing a mixture of anesthesia and oxygen. With facial surgery, many anesthetists will insert a tube in the trachea (entubation) to maintain the anesthesia as well as to ensure that you breath properly. Entubation is not usually necessary for such procedures as liposuction or breast surgeries. You may wake up with a temporary sore throat if you have been entubated.

In the past, many doctors administered their own anesthesia. Anesthetists even carried their own equipment around with them because doctors' offices were insufficiently equipped. The best outpatient facilities are set up as adequately as a hospital operating room, but unfortunately, with the lack of legislation, many outpatient facilities are still under-equipped for emergencies or even adequate care. Until these facilities are regulated by the government, many will probably continue in this condition. Some doctors use staff that have not been properly trained in the administration of anesthesia, monitoring of patients, or in emergency techniques. A cosmetic surgery candidate should be deeply concerned with finding out that their surgeon employs the appropriate staff and that emergency medications are on hand. In the world of unregulated outpatient facilities, one cannot afford to be less than fanatical.

FACELIFT
RHYTIDECTOMY

Rhytidectomy typically is performed to remove excess or loose, sagging skin from the face and neck. . . . When removal of pouches around the eyes is desirable, eyelid surgery, or blepharoplasty, may be done in conjunction with the facelift operation or as a separate procedure.

Rhytidectomy may be performed under a local anesthetic which numbs the area to be treated or a general anesthetic may be used. . . .

Rhytidectomy is performed first on one side of the face and then the other. Some of the hairline will be shaved before incisions are made. Incisions frequently are individualized to fit the patient's needs and the surgeon's methods. In most cases an incision is started inside the hairline at the temples, continues downward in a natural line around the earlobe and extends into the back of the scalp or nape of the neck. Occasionally an incision may extend inside the front of the ear. A small incision frequently is necessary under the chin to provide access to excess neck skin.

Working through the incision, the surgeon separates the skin from underlying fat and muscle. The skin is pulled up and

Courtesy of the American Society of Plastic and Reconstructive Surgeons.

backward in the temple area, as well as in the front and back of the ear, and the excess is excised. In some cases, accumulations of fat are removed from beneath the chin and neck, and sagging muscles and connective tissues are tightened.

If blepharoplasty is to be performed during the same operation, the surgeon will make incisions on the upper and lower eyelids, generally extending into the "crow's feet" at the outer edge of the eyes. Subsequently excess skin and underlying fat will be removed.

Sutures close the incisions along the natural skin lines and creases. Although the surgeon has made every effort to keep scars as inconspicuous as possible, they are the inevitable result of surgery. In most patients scars will fade gradually and become barely visible. Those that are most noticeable, in back of the ear, can be covered conveniently by the individual's hair. Following surgery, a small thin tube may be placed in the back of the ear to allow drainage of any blood collecting under the skin. Large loose dressings will be applied to the face and neck. Depending on the extent of the surgery, with or without blepharoplasty, the procedure usually lasts from two to four hours or longer.

After surgery . . . you will be asked to keep your head slightly elevated for a few days. If a drain has been inserted, it will be removed in a day or two following the operation. Dressings commonly are removed in a few days. A patient who was admitted to a hospital will be released in two to four days. Swelling and skin discoloration are common and usually will subside within a week or two. Many patients report a sense of tightness or numbness of the face and neck after surgery. The intensity of these conditions and how long they will last varies with the individual.

The objective of a facelift operation is a natural, younger, more attractive appearance. However, normal healing is a gradual process, with final results not fully realized for at least three weeks.

THE DEEP-PLANE
RHYTIDECTOMY

Some surgeons have adopted a relatively new facelift technique presented first at the Annual Meeting of the American Society for Aesthetic Plastic Surgery in San Francisco in March, 1988, by Dr. Sam Hamra of Dallas, Texas. The technique, "deep-plane" rhytidectomy, involves a dissection exactly like it sounds: instead of merely separating the skin and pulling it back, the surgeon extends the cut through the subcutaneous fatty layer and through the muscle, moving the entire mass up and back to where it was before gravity and age took over. The biggest advantage of this procedure shows in the "nasolabial folds," which are the vertical creases that run down from the outer edges of the nostrils to the corners of the mouth. With the old techniques, very little improvement in the nasolabial folds can be discerned. After a deep-plane rhytidectomy, the improvement is remarkable.

FOREHEAD LIFT

A forehead lift is most often used to improve such facial characteristics as drooping eyebrows, "hooding" or drooping tissue at the outer part of the eyes, furrowed forehead and frown lines at the top of the nose. The desired result is a more alert and less tired appearance, smoother forehead skin and softer lines between the eyes. Often, a forehead lift is performed in conjunction with a facelift.

. . .

The surgery may take one to two hours. Unless you have a high or receding hairline, an incision will be made across the top of your head a few inches behind your hairline to minimize the possibility of the scar being visible. If you *do* have a high or receding hairline, the incision will be made at the hairline, in which case a thin line may be visible and may need to be covered with your hair.

The purpose of the operation is to interrupt the downward pull of the muscles that cause facial features to droop. This is accomplished by removing several strips of your forehead muscle. Most plastic surgeons feel that removal of this muscle

Courtesy of the American Society of Plastic and Reconstructive Surgeons.

tissue helps maintain the lift and gives you a longer-lasting result. In addition, if you have deep, vertical furrows at the top of your nose, your surgeon will remove a portion of the muscles between the eyebrows.

When these steps are completed, the forehead skin [flap] will be gently pulled upward, and any excess skin at the point of incision will be removed. The surgeon will close the incision with a series of stitches or staples, wash your face and hair to prevent irritation, and remove the bands from your hair. Gauze padding will be placed across the incision, and your head will be wrapped with a stretch or elastic bandage.

Following surgery, you may feel some temporary pain that can be controlled with medication. . . . Some bruising and swelling are natural, and will begin to decrease in a week to 10 days. . . .

Bandages will be removed one or two days following surgery. Stitches or staples used to close the incision will be removed in 10 days to two weeks following surgery. . . .

Most patients begin to resume their normal routines very quickly following a forehead lift, usually within a week after surgery. Generally, they are back to work within a week to 10 days. . . .

You will be able to wash your hair one or two days after surgery. . . .

[Editor's note: In a forehead lift, there will always be a loss of sensation above the scar because the nerves for the forehead come out of the skull at the eyebrows and run upwards. These nerves are severed at surgery, and the result is a permanent loss of feeling between the scar and the middle of the head. Too much tension on the flap of forehead skin, or slicing the flap too thin, can cause thinning of the hair in front of the incision. Hair loss on the rest of the head has been noted, but the reason for such loss is undetermined—KO]

EYELID SURGERY
BLEPHAROPLASTY

Blepharoplasty typically is performed to remove excess folds of skin, pouches under the eyes and, in some instances, is accompanied by an additional procedure to correct sagging eyebrows. One or all of these changes can be made during a single operation. . . .

. . . you may be operated on in the surgeon's office, in an outpatient surgical facility or you may be admitted to a hospital. Blepharoplasty may be performed under a local anesthetic which numbs the area to be treated or a general anesthetic may be used. . . .

Blepharoplasty usually is performed first on the upper lid and then the lower. In both areas, underlying compartments of fat will be removed. Incisions in the upper and lower eyelids are made following natural lines and creases, and generally extend into the first wrinkling, or crow's feet, at the eyes' outer edge. Working through the incisions, the surgeon separates skin from underlying fatty tissue and muscle. Exposed fat and excess skin are removed.

The number and type of sutures used to close the incisions

vary, depending on the surgeon's judgment. Once healed, the hairline scars will fade and become barely visible within six to eight weeks.

Following surgery, moist gauze dressings will be applied to the eyes.

Depending on the extent of the surgery, the procedure usually lasts from one to two hours or longer.

After surgery, there is some soreness and discomfort. . . . You will be asked to keep your head slightly elevated and apply cold compresses to your eyes to help reduce swelling and bruising. If dressings are applied they are usually removed on the eve of surgery or on the following day.

You will be instructed to rinse your eyes with an eye wash and to use eye drops for several days following surgery.

Eyelid skin, being thin, tends to swell and discolor rapidly after surgery. However, when sutures are removed within a week of surgery, swelling and black-and-blue discoloration will subside. Residual bruising can be covered by light makeup. Other postoperative effects of short duration may include excessive tearing and sensitivity to bright light.

. . .

Wearing of dark glasses to protect the eyes from wind and sun irritation is suggested for two to three weeks.

SURGERY OF THE NOSE
Rhinoplasty

Aesthetic rhinoplasty typically is performed to reduce the overall size of the nose, reshape a tip, remove a nasal hump or improve a poor angle between the nose and the upper lip. In some patients it is necessary to add tissue in order to improve contour. One or all of these changes can be made during a single operation. . . .

In most nasal surgery an incision is made inside the nostrils, through which the work will be done. The incision provides the surgeon with access to cartilage and bone which can be cut, trimmed and manipulated to reshape the nose and alter its external appearance.

A hump is removed by using a sawing instrument or a chisel and then bringing the nasal bones together to form a narrower bridge. Removing the cartilage reduces the size of the nasal tip and provides better contour. To improve the angle between the bottom portion of the nose and the upper lip, the nasal tip is elevated. This is accomplished by trimming the septum through the incisions in the nostrils. If a large hump is removed, the base of the nose is disproportionately wide. To

Courtesy of the American Society of Plastic and Reconstructive Surgeons.

narrow it, small skin wedges are removed and the nostrils are brought closer to the center. Following surgery, a splint composed of tape and a plastic or plaster overlay is applied to the nose to maintain bone and cartilage in their new shape. Frequently nasal packs are inserted to protect the nasal septum, particularly if septal surgery has been performed.

The procedure usually lasts from an hour and a half to two hours or longer, depending on the extent of the surgery.

After the operation, there is some pain. . . . You will be asked to keep your head slightly elevated and apply cold compresses to your eyes to reduce postoperative bruising and swelling.

The splint is often removed within a week of surgery, although it may remain in place for up to ten days. Your surgeon may advise you to wear the splint at night. Nasal packing may stay in a few days before it is removed. Bruising around the eyes will begin to fade within a few days following the operation and will generally disappear within the next two to three weeks. Subtle swelling of the nose subsides gradually; some swelling may be present for months.

. . .

It is common after some types of rhinoplasty for relatives or friends to remark that they do not see a major difference. Do not consider such a reaction an indication of failure. On the contrary, if it looks *better* and *natural,* it may go unnoticed. The intention, after all, is not to create a "new" nose that draws attention to itself, but rather one that blends subtly into the overall features of the face in the proper proportions.

CHIN AUGMENTATION
GENIOPLASTY
(MENTOPLASTY)

Aesthetic genioplasty typically is performed to add size and contour to a receding chin. The patient usually has a normal bite, or dental occlusion, which will not be affected by chin augmentation. . . .

Genioplasty usually is performed under a local anesthetic which numbs the area around the chin. . . .

There are two basic approaches to genioplasty. In some cases it may be best to move the chin bone. In this technique, the surgeon makes an incision inside the mouth to gain access to the chin bone. Using a sawing instrument or chisel, the surgeon makes a horizontal cut through the bone. The lower portion of the separated bone is moved forward and wired in position. The incision in the mouth is closed with sutures and an external pressure dressing is generally placed over the chin. Since surgery is performed through an internal incision, the patient has no visible scarring.

When only a modest degree of chin augmentation is required to provide contour, the surgeon may use a plastic chin implant, or prosthesis. In this technique, the incision is made

Courtesy of the American Society of Plastic and Reconstructive Surgeons.

either inside the mouth or externally on the underside of the chin. Working through the incision, the surgeon creates a pocket above the chin bone and under the muscles, and inserts an appropriately-sized prosthesis or chin implant. The incision is closed and a pressure dressing is applied. The resultant scar from the external incision is negligible.

. . . The patient is generally up and about the same day as surgery and back to work and normal activities within a few days. The dressing usually is removed within a week of surgery.

CHEMICAL PEEL
CHEMOSURGERY

Chemosurgery typically is performed to improve fine wrinkling over the forehead, about the eyelids and cheeks, and around the mouth. . . .

Before surgery, you will be given medication to alleviate tension and relieve discomfort that may occur during the procedure.

In chemosurgery, a chemical solution is applied to the areas to be treated. In a chemical peel of the entire face, the liquid is applied to all areas except eyes, brows and lips. For many chemosurgery patients, the mouth is the only area treated. It can be done alone or in conjunction with a facelift operation. However, a full face peel cannot be done when a facelift has been performed.

A burning sensation may be experienced when the solution is applied, but should pass quickly as the chemical itself acts as a local anesthetic.

When performing chemical peel to minimize wrinkles, the surgeon usually will cover the face with a "mask" composed of strips of adhesive tape with openings for the eyes and mouth.

Courtesy of the American Society of Plastic and Reconstructive Surgeons.

When the peel is done primarily for skin blemishes or pigmentation problems, tape may not be used.

Depending on the extent of the surgery, the procedure usually lasts for one hour or longer.

After surgery, there is some discomfort that is controlled by medication. Abnormal sensations, such as itching and tingling, may be experienced as the skin heals. These sensations can be alleviated with cold compresses and appropriate medication.

If a mask has been used, it will be removed a day or two after chemosurgery. A crust or scab to protect the new skin will develop over the areas treated within twenty-four hours. It is removed by gentle cleansing with soap and water, and the application of ointments, creams, or moisturizers. A patient who was admitted to a hospital will be released at this time.

Following removal of the crust, the exposed skin layer will take on a deep red color, not unlike a severe sunburn. This will gradually turn to a pinkish hue. When the new skin has been regenerated completely after several weeks, it will permanently be a bit lighter in color than it was before the surgery. Tiny whiteheads, or milia, may appear and usually can be washed away with a soapy cloth. Stubborn cases can be treated quickly by the surgeon.

After chemosurgery, the patient will have tighter, smoother skin that is relatively free of blemishes and wrinkles in the areas treated. There will be improvement in the skin as evidenced by a younger, fresher appearance of the face. Swelling and puffing out of fine lines and wrinkles shortly after surgery may show more dramatic results than is the case when final healing is complete. Fine lines may reappear as the swelling subsides, but they will not be as prominent as before chemosurgery. Exposure to direct sunlight should be avoided completely for the first three weeks to prevent uneven skin tone. Skin pores may be a little larger following surgery. The skin is generally not able to tan smoothly following chemosurgery, therefore, it should be protected from prolonged exposure to the sun. Light exposure is permitted for the next several months only when the patient wears a sun blocking cream.

[Editor's note: A phenol peel should be applied to very small areas at a time. Inhalation of the chemicals involved can cause cardiac arrhythmia in a high percentage of cases where caution is not observed. Some anesthesiologists recommend entubation during a chemical peel, which is the insertion of a tube into the trachea so that the patient breathes with the assistance of an oxygen machine, thus avoiding inhalation of the fumes and the resultant problems—KO]

A WARNING FROM THE FDA REGARDING CHEMICAL PEELS

From *FDA Backgrounder*
MAY 21, 1992

The Food and Drug Administration today cautioned consumers about possible hazards associated with use of chemical skin peeling products. The agency also has begun an investigation to determine the seriousness of injuries reported to be associated with such products and the extent to which they occur.

"We are warning consumers about the use of skin peelers because they can cause serious injuries, particularly when not used under the supervision of a physician," said Commissioner David A. Kessler, M.D.

FDA issued the warning after it received reports of several injuries caused by skin peelers including four reports of skin burns from using a product called PeelAway. The agency said there may be other unreported injuries from PeelAway, as well as from other skin peeling products.

The products in question contain ingredients that purportedly remove wrinkles, blemishes, blotches and acne scars. They are often promoted with claims that they can restore youthful-looking skin.

FDA said such products can penetrate the skin too deeply, causing severe skin damage. In several cases, persons have been hospitalized for severe burns, swelling and pain. In one case, a California woman suffered seizure, shock and second degree burns after a mixture of skin peel chemicals was applied to her legs by a beautician. The case is under review by California state health officials.

Skin peeling products vary considerably as to their ingredients and strength. Also, skin reactions to the chemicals used in the products vary among individuals. Skin peeling products typically contain combinations and concentrations of several different acids such as resorcinol, phenol, lactic acid, trichloroacetic acid, salicylic acid, and glycolic acid and other alphahydroxy acids.

They are ordinarily applied to the skin for a short time each day, usually for six to 12 days. The skin initially reddens, as with a sunburn, then darkens and finally peels away revealing what manufacturers claim will be "new skin." Treatments may be painful and leave permanent scars.

Skin peeling procedures used to be carried out only by plastic surgeons and dermatologists. However, they are now being done by a variety of non-medical professionals such as cosmetologists and beauticians, some using newly marketed preparations. Several of the products can be purchased through the mail. Many have inadequate instructions; *none have been approved as being safe and effective.*

In the course of conducting its investigation, FDA will review all products marketed with skin peeling claims. Dr. Kessler said FDA is working with state attorneys general who are also taking measures to stop the sale and use of hazardous skin peeling products.

In a warning letter sent to PeelAway manufacturer Global Esthetics of Seattle, Wash., May 14, FDA said that it considers PeelAway to be a new drug that cannot be legally marketed without FDA approval, and that the product is misbranded and presents a significant health hazard.

The actions being announced now are not directed at facial mask-type products intended for one-time or occasional use to cleanse the skin.

BREAST AUGMENTATION
AUGMENTATION MAMMOPLASTY

During the initial visit, the surgeon will explain specific details of your case, including the surgical technique to be used, the anesthesia, where the operation will be performed and what the surgery realistically can accomplish. Additional factors to consider before electing augmentation mammoplasty, such as risk and cost, should be discussed with the surgeon at this time.

After examining you, the surgeon will discuss . . . variables that influence the decisions involved in the procedure, such as condition of the breast and skin on the chest wall cavity. For patients with marked sagging of the breasts, the surgeon may recommend a procedure to reduce and reshape breast skin in addition to augmentation mammoplasty.

Postoperative complications such as infection or localized collections of blood are uncommon and can be treated. Occasionally a second operation may be required to soften breasts that become too firm due to excessive scar tissue formation called capsular contracture.

Fees and operative facility costs of augmentation

Courtesy of the American Society of Plastic and Reconstructive Surgeons.

mammoplasty vary widely. A recent study that surveyed member surgeons [of the ASPRS], and the hospitals with which they are affiliated, determined total surgical fees range from $2,000 to $3,000 or more, depending on the length and complexity of the operation. Additional expenses will depend upon the anesthesia used and where the operation takes place.

Augmentation mammoplasty typically is performed to enlarge small, underdeveloped breasts or breasts that have decreased in size after childbearing. It may also be done to balance asymmetry. . . .

There are several possible approaches to breast augmentation. The most commonly employed techniques are an inframammary incision which is made slightly above where the lower part of the breast touches the chest, or a periareolar incision which is made around the lower border of the areola, the dark pink skin that surrounds the nipple. Another less frequently used approach is an axilla incision made in the armpit. The surgical technique employed will depend on the surgeon's preference.

Working through the incision, the surgeon lifts breast tissue up and skin down to create a pocket either directly under the tissue or underneath the chest wall muscle, depending on the surgeon's technique and the patient's anatomy. In the pocket the surgeon places a breast implant, or prosthesis, which is a flexible plastic envelope containing . . . saline solution. A few sutures close the incision.

Following surgery, a gauze dressing may be applied over the breasts, or the patient may be placed in a surgical bra.

Depending on the extent of the surgery, the procedure usually lasts about two hours or longer.

After surgery, pain that is easily controlled by medication usually will subside in a day or two. If you have been admitted to a hospital, you will be released within a couple of days following the operation.

If dressings have been applied, they will be replaced by a surgical bra in a few days. Sutures will be removed within a week of surgery. Although the surgeon has made every effort to keep scars as inconspicuous as possible, they are the inevitable result of surgery. In most cases, they will begin to fade gradually and become barely noticeable. Minimal swelling and discoloration of the breasts will disappear rapidly.

The objective of augmentation mammoplasty is breasts that look fuller and more natural in appearance.

Asymmetry of the breasts may result from a difference in the healing process on the two sides. Some degree of firmness of the breasts may occur for weeks or even months following surgery. In some instances, the surgeon may recommend a program of breast massage to promote softness. There may be a loss of sensitivity in the nipples following the operation, but in most cases a degree of sensitivity will return.

Although you may be up and about in a day or two following surgery, your plastic surgeon will advise you on the proper schedule for resuming your normal routine. To permit proper healing, you should avoid overactivity and refrain from overhead lifting. . . .

BREAST LIFT
MASTOPEXY

The surgeon will conduct a routine breast examination and, depending on your age and family history, may determine that mammograms, or breast x-rays, are required. After examining you, the surgeon will discuss other variables that influence the decisions involved in the procedure, such as your age, the size and shape of your breasts and the condition of breast skin. A patient considering breast-feeding following mastopexy should discuss the matter with the plastic surgeon at this time.

Mastopexy typically is performed to lift sagging, loose breasts or breasts that have lost volume and elasticity after childbearing. It also can reduce the size of the areola, the dark pink skin surrounding the nipple. . . .

You may be operated on in the surgeon's office, in an outpatient surgical facility or you may be admitted to a hospital. Mastopexy usually is performed under general anesthesia to make you sleep through the entire operation, although local anesthesia to numb the area around the breasts may be used. . . .

In the operation, the surgeon makes incisions following the natural contour across the breast and around the areola. A

Courtesy of the American Society of Plastic and Reconstructive Surgeons.

keyhole-shaped incision also is made above the areola to define the new location for the nipple.

Working through the horizontal incisions, the surgeon removes excess skin from the lower section of the breast. The nipple, areola and underlying breast tissue are moved up to a new higher position. After the nipple is relocated, flaps of skin formerly above and to the sides of the nipple are brought down, around and together to reshape the breast. Sutures close the wounds under the breast and around the nipple area.

In patients with only minimal sagging, a modified procedure may be used to excise only skin from the large areola and the area immediately surrounding it.

Depending on the extent of the surgery, the procedure usually lasts about two hours.

Following surgery, a bulky gauze dressing is wrapped around the breasts, or the patient may be wrapped in a surgical bra. . . . Within the first week, the dressing will be replaced by a soft bra which you will be advised to wear for several weeks.

Swelling and discoloration around the incisions generally will subside in a few days. After surgery, there may be temporary loss of sensation in the nipples and breast skin. If it occurs, this condition will improve with time. Sutures will be removed within two weeks of surgery.

The objective of mastopexy is higher, well-contoured breasts. Although the surgeon makes every effort to keep scars as inconspicuous as possible, mastopexy scars are permanent. They often remain highly visible for a year following surgery, then fade to some degree. However, since incisions are made around and below the nipples, scars should not be noticeable even in low-cut clothing.

BREAST REDUCTION
REDUCTION MAMMOPLASTY

Women with disproportionately large, sagging breasts are good candidates for breast reduction. Those who have breasts that sag but are not too large might benefit more from a breast lift (mastopexy).

While women of any age can benefit from the procedure, it usually is performed after breasts are fully developed unless a young girl experiences great physical discomfort due to the size of her breasts.

Breast reduction is not recommended for women who want to breastfeed. The ability to breastfeed cannot be predicted following the procedure since ducts leading to and from the nipple may have to be severed to achieve the reduction.

Breast reduction does leave scars under the breasts and leading up to the nipple, although they lighten to some extent with time. Minor surgery can improve scars that are very visible, but they cannot be erased. Sometimes sensitivity in the nipple and breast is reduced, and feeling may not return for as long as six months.

Because blood transfusions may be required during sur-

Courtesy of the American Society of Plastic and Reconstructive Surgeons.

gery, particularly if you have very large breasts, you may want to talk with your doctor about having blood drawn and "banked" prior to surgery.

The surgery will take three to four hours, depending on the extent of the procedure. Generally, incisions are made horizontally and vertically following the natural contour of the breast. The vertical incision creates a key-hole-shaped pattern around the areola to allow the nipple to be repositioned. Excess tissue, fat and skin are removed from the sides of the breast and around the areola. Then the nipple, areola and underlying tissue are moved to a new, higher location. If breasts are extremely large, the surgeon may completely detach the nipple before it is relocated.

When the nipple is repositioned, skin on both sides of the breast is moved down and around the areola and brought together to reform the breast. The incision will be closed with stitches under the breast and around the nipple. A gauze dressing may be applied or a surgical bra may be fitted.

Within a week, any surgical dressing will be replaced with a soft bra, which you will be asked to wear for several weeks. Swelling and skin discoloration around the incisions usually will subside in a few days, and stitches will be removed in two to three weeks.

TUMMY TUCK
ABDOMINOPLASTY

Abdominoplasty typically is performed to remove excess abdominal skin and tighten underlying musculature. The extent of the procedure depends on what changes are desired and what your surgeon deems appropriate. Abdominoplasty usually is performed in a hospital under general anesthesia.

There are several possible approaches to abdominoplasty. The most frequently employed technique is a transverse incision across the lower abdomen, just above the pubic area. A second incision is made to free the umbilicus from the surrounding skin so it will remain undisturbed. Skin is separated from the abdominal wall and elevated above the rib cage. The surgeon then pulls loose tissue covering the abdomen's large vertical muscle towards the center of the abdomen and sutures it together. This tightens muscles, provides a firmer abdominal wall and narrows the waistline. The elevated skin is lowered and the excess removed. The surgeon makes a small opening for the umbilicus. It is reinstated, creating a new navel where the old one had been. Incisions are closed with a series of stitches and a firm elastic dressing is applied.

Courtesy of the American Society of Plastic and Reconstructive Surgeons.

After surgery, there is soreness and discomfort which is easily controlled by medication.

The patient will remain in the hospital for two to three days with hips bent to reduce tension on the abdominal area. The dressing is replaced by an appropriate abdominal supporter before the patient is discharged. He or she is advised to continue wearing a light support garment for two to three months.

[Editor's Note: Tummy tucks are frequently performed in out-patient clinics. From the description of the procedure, the reader will note that this is truly major surgery. Use caution when considering this procedure in an outpatient setting—KO]

LIPOSUCTION
BODY FAT REDUCTION OR SUCTION-ASSISTED LIPECTOMY

Suction-assisted lipectomy—liposuction—is not a substitute for weight reduction that can be attained through dieting and exercise, nor is it a cure for obesity. It is a surgical technique suitable for carefully selected patients. Your surgeon may recommend surgical lipectomy, in which excess skin and fat are removed, instead of, or in addition to, suction-assisted lipectomy.

Suction-assisted lipectomy typically is performed on a patient of relatively normal body build and weight to reduce disproportionately large hips, buttocks and thighs, a protruding abdomen or "love handles" above the waist. These changes, as well as removal of fat on arms, calves, and knees, above the breasts and under the chin, often can be made during a single operation. . . .

Surgery begins with incisions of about one-half-inch in length made in the area where suction-assisted lipectomy will be performed. A blunt-ended tubular instrument with an opening near the end is passed through the incisions. A suction unit is attached to the protruding end. The surgeon manipulates the instrument in the tissue under the skin, separating the amount

Courtesy of the American Society of Plastic and Reconstructive Surgeons.

of fat to be removed. High vacuum pressure is created and the fat is suctioned off.

Occasionally an additional incision is required to gain access to all unwanted fat deposits to be removed.

A few sutures close the incisions leaving small and often concealed scars.

Following surgery, a snug dressing of elastic gauze may be applied over the entire treated area to promote skin shrinkage to conform smoothly to the shape of the underlying tissue. In some instances, a long-length corset-like garment is used to secure firm compression to the area to reduce swelling and skin discoloration.

Depending on the extent of the surgery, the procedure usually lasts from 45 minutes to two hours or longer.

After surgery, pain that can be controlled by medication may be present for several days. Numbness or discomfort may be experienced for varying periods of time.

A patient who was admitted to a hospital will be released two or three days following the operation. The protective bandages or corset-like garment often are removed within a week of surgery. However, to further proper skin shrinkage, you may be asked to wear a long-legged girdle for two to three months.

Some swelling and skin discoloration will exist, but usually will subside within six to eight weeks. There is a possibility that skin over the treated area will have a rippled or uneven effect. If surface imperfections such as skin dimpling (often called cellulite) are present before surgery, they will remain after it. In some cases, permanent sagging of the skin may occur when the fat removed from the area exceeds the capacity of the skin to contract.

Patients with localized deposits of fat, who are also over-weight, must be willing to accept a greater possibility of contour irregularities and poor skin redraping in exchange for looking better in clothing. An older individual with loss of skin elasticity may require surgical removal of excess skin as a secondary procedure to achieve maximum results.

[Editor's note: Doctors are able to remove larger amounts of fat in one procedure than previously. However, 1500 cubic centimeters is considered a safe amount to remove without a blood transfusion. If you are having liposuction performed on your hips and thighs and you have a considerable amount of fat to be removed, you should have a unit of your own blood drawn and banked prior to surgery for a transfusion. Ask your surgeon what he or she suggests—KO]

A SHORT LESSON IN LIPOSUCTION

by Elizabeth Karlsberg

"Cosmetic Surgery Update"
Teen
January 1991

When done properly by a qualified surgeon, liposuction works quite well at removing localized pockets of fat cells. . . . [Doctors] emphasize that liposuction is not a treatment for obesity. It's for those people who have an out-of-proportion fat deposit—which usually means in the "riding breeches area" of the thigh, the hips or the lower belly. (Fat cells can also be removed from other areas, such as the knees and the upper front of the neck; although for teens, the other areas are more common.)

As Dr. [Gregory] Wingate [of Phoenix, Arizona,] explains, "A person is born with a finite number of fat cells. Throughout life, these fat cells are either filled up and made larger or made smaller through dieting. So where you have an area of fatty fullness in a young person, you have an increased number of fat cells at that site."

The ideal liposuction candidate, therefore, is a person with young, elastic skin who is not overweight, but rather has localized collections of fat. In fact, many liposuction patients are quite fit and trim, and yet they still have these areas of pudge that just won't budge. Losing more weight isn't the answer, particularly when a person is already at her ideal weight, since these places are always the very last to go.

What happens if you gain weight after liposuction? Will you once again deposit more fat in the same areas from which fat was removed?

"You can definitely gain weight," says Dr. Wingate, "but you will probably never gain weight proportionally to that area. Since we don't remove all that many fat cells from an area, you can still gain fullness there, but never to the same extent that you would have had had you not had liposuction."

A GROWTH INDUSTRY IN CHINA
PENILE AUGMENTATION

By Lena H. Sun

Washington Post Foreign Service
Washington Post
November 17, 1991

W UHAN, China—Every month, surgeon Long Daochou receives hundreds of letters from Chinese men who want his help in saving their marriages, restoring their self-esteem and preserving the family line.

As his fame spreads, the demand for his service has intensified. Every day, 10 or more prospective patients await him at his hospital, to plead for his knife.

He has become one of the most famous practitioners in China because he has resurrected an ancient procedure that can make penises longer.

Among men everywhere, genital size has always been the stuff of crude jokes and locker room banter. But in China—particularly recently—it has become something of a national obsession. Men are willing to go to great lengths, as it were, for greater length.

In one typical Chinese department store in Beijing, out in the open next to shoe brushes, cigarette lighters and incense sticks, is a display case of assorted stretchers and puffers and vacuum-pump contraptions said to increase penis length and girth. They sell briskly. Most of them are stupid doodads that don't work.

Long's surgery seems to.

Long says the simple technique can lengthen a penis by as much as two inches without affecting sensitivity or function. When two ligaments are cut that attach the penis to the pubic bone, he says, an internal portion of the penis is extended out of the body. The whole process takes about 90 minutes and can be performed using general or local anesthesia. Full recovery takes about a month.

Although some Western practitioners are skeptical about the procedure and worry about its side effects, "we have not had a single failure yet," Long said, referring to the 218 operations he has performed since 1984—about half of them in the past year alone.

Long is chief of the plastic surgery department at the First Affiliated Hospital of the Hubei Medical College here in this industrial city in central China. He's the only doctor in China doing the operation, and now he's doing as many as four a week. He can barely keep up with the demand.

Long will take as patients only men with real problems— not normally proportioned men who want to feel like studs.

"This abnormal illness has made our sexual relations bad," wrote a 40-year-old factory worker with an abnormally small organ. "Because of this, we are often unhappy. If you can cure this illness, I will regain my wife's love."

Long took the case.

One young man who graduated from college in 1984 fears he will never be able to get married because his penis is only three centimeters, or a bit more than an inch long, flaccid.

"Because of this, I dare not wash in public. . . . My college classmates are already fathers, but I don't dare to look for girlfriends even though there are many girls chasing me," he wrote. "I am in deep pain and I feel like killing myself."

Even though Long claims he invented the technique, the procedure is described in some detail in the Kamasutra, the

Indian epic about eroticism that dates back to A.D. 300.

The operation costs between 800 and 1,000 yuan, or about $149 to $186, cheap by Western standards but exorbitant for working-class Chinese, whose average monthly salary may be 150 yuan. The operation is not covered under state medical insurance, and patients often have to borrow money from relatives and friends, Long said. (Like most doctors in China, Long draws a fixed salary and does not receive any extra money from the operations.)

In the United States, although some plastic surgeons offer penis-thickening operations (the procedure is more or less the opposite of liposuction), Long's surgery is rarely if ever performed. Ricardo Samitier, a Miami physician, offers only the fattening operation. He call's Long's procedure "just an optical illusion," since no additional flesh is added to the organ. He said it is like "saying you are making a building taller by exposing its foundation."

Other Western experts express different reservations. The operation can harm the nerves that go to the penis and, over the long term, might make it shorter rather than longer, says Ira Goldstein, a urologist at the Boston University School of Medicine.

"But I guess the question is," he said, "would a man offered a chance to have one-hour outpatient surgery to lengthen his penis be interested?"

Well . . . yes.

[Editor's note: Why hasn't this procedure been pursued more avidly in this country? After all, women have been augmenting their breasts for thirty years—KO]

LASER SURGERY

The word "laser" symbolizes advanced technology. Laser surgery: the knife that isn't a knife but a Star Trek force field able to cut without blood. How much does the layman understand about lasers? Probably not much.

Lasers work by burning through tissue, and cauterizing the wound as they cut. Therefore, less bleeding is encountered during a procedure. However, many doctors remain unconvinced of their value as a precision cutting tool.

According to one doctor from Newport Beach, California, the major benefit of a laser is in its marketing value; it sounds like mystical science fiction and "it has a lot of sex appeal." Dr. Lawrence Seifert of Beverly Hills agrees. "For many people, the implication that there's a laser involved indicates a certainty in precision of the results. That enables the practitioner who markets it that way to unconsciously prey on a lack of sophistication in science by the consumer of our services. They may think that because a laser is used, they're going to have a superior result, and so, 'I know my eyelids are going to look great!' And there's never been a single article in my mind in our literature where it's been shown that the use of a laser is beneficial for standard aesthetic operations, including facelifts."

Studies have shown little difference in the results of surgery using a laser and surgery using a cold, sharp knife. According to a 1990 study by Drs. Harry Mittelman of Palo Alto and David Apfelberg of Atherton, California, lasers may produce less bleeding during the surgery than an ordinary 50-cent scalpel, but the results of the surgery are basically the same. Lasers, on the other hand, are extremely expensive tools—they can run as much as a quarter of a million dollars, and that's a lot of face lifts. Lasers also require trained support personnel, special equipment such as goggles and gloves, and additional storage space. Lasers eject a smoke plume when in use that must be removed with yet another special piece of equipment. Who bears the cost of this "improved" technique? The patients who have been enticed into the surgeon's office with the promise of "state of the art" techniques—that's who.

A laser can do a great deal of harm in the hands of an inexperienced practitioner. Since lasers work by burning tissue, a too-long or too-strong exposure can literally burn holes through the skin (they're called "buttonholes"). In eyelid surgery, a common use for lasers, a few millimeters the wrong way can puncture the globe of the eye. When the eye is punctured, the *aquaeous humor* which it contains and which maintains the round shape leaks out, causing the eyeball to detach from the retina. Result: blindness.

Notwithstanding the dangers and problems with laser-assisted cosmetic surgery, the future holds promise. Researchers such as Dr. Apfelberg continue to explore new uses for lasers. A new type of cannula for liposuction using laser, for example, is being tested by the FDA. With this technique, the laser cauterizes the area as fat is suctioned out through the cannula, allowing the doctor to remove much more fat without the necessity of a blood transfusion. "Laser resurfacing," a laser-assisted peel, burns off the outer layer of the skin just as a chemical peel would. Dr. Laurence David of Hermosa Beach,

California, offers this service. The recovery time is one to two weeks as opposed to several months with the chemical procedure. The cost: as much as eight times that of a chemical peel.

With all new or experimental techniques, the costs and the risks are high. Lasers definitely present an exciting future, and certainly bear watching. But caution is advisable when considering laser-assisted cosmetic surgery: maybe you can buy the *Starship Enterprise*, but do you know how to drive it?

COLLAGEN AND LIQUID SILICONE INJECTIONS

from FDA Backgrounder: Current and Useful Information from the Food & Drug Administration

The following information has been prepared by the Food and Drug Administration to answer questions about the regulatory status and the possible risks of two cosmetic procedures: collagen injections and silicone injections. FDA has approved collagen injections for some purposes; it has not approved silicone injections for *any* purposes.

INJECTABLE COLLAGEN

1) **What is injectable collagen?** Injectable collagen is a liquid made from the connective tissue of cows or pigs that is injected into and under the skin for cosmetic purposes. Two trade names for the type derived from cows are Zyderm and Zyplast, both manufactured by the Collagen Corporation. Another product, manufactured from pig collagen by Mentor Corporation, is known as Fibrel.

2) **What are the FDA-approved uses for injectable collagen?** Injectable collagen has been approved by FDA for filling in "contour deformities" in the skin such as

acne scars and wrinkles. It is *not* approved for "aug-mentation" - that is, enlarging otherwise normal facial features. It is also not approved for injection directly into the pigmented area of the lips (but it can be used to correct wrinkles on the skin bordering the lips).

3) **How long do the effects of treatment last?** To main-tain the effect, collagen injections are usually repeated periodically. The time between treatments varies de-pending on the patient and the part of the face being treated. Generally, the effects of treatment last from a few months to about a year and a half. In some cases, the effects are shorter-lasting, whereas in others they have been known to last two years or longer.

4) **What are the risks of collagen treatments?** About three percent of the population is allergic to collagen, and these people should not receive the treatments. (This includes individuals who have had allergic reactions to other collagen-containing products, such as surgical sutures and sponges.) Collagen injections should also not be given to people with severe allergies to numer-ous other substances.

People may be allergic to collagen and not know it. For this reason, all patients considering collagen injections **must** first be tested for collagen allergy. To do this, the doctor injects a small amount of collagen in the forearm and watches for a reaction for four weeks before begin-ning any treatment. Even the allergy test is not perfect—a small percentage of patients who do not react to the test have developed allergies during the course of treatment.

Collagen allergies can take the form of rash, hives, joint and muscle pain, headache, and, in a few cases, severe reactions that include shock and difficulty breathing. Other adverse effects that have occurred after collagen injections, and which appear to have been related to the injections, include infections, abscesses, open sores, lumps, peeling of the skin, scarring, recurrence of herpes simplex, and partial blindness.

Patients with certain connective diseases may have an increased risk of severe allergic reactions to collagen injections. These connective tissue diseases include, but are not limited to, rheumatoid arthritis, scleroderma, and juvenile rheumatoid arthritis. They also include polymyositis and dermatomyositis ('PM/DM"), which are chronic, progressive, sometimes fatal inflammatory disorders. Thus, collagen injections should be used with caution in people who have had these diseases. Some experts recommend that people who have had these diseases should either not be given collagen injections at all or should be given multiple skin tests before treatment.

Some physicians have reported that patients developed PM/DM and other connective tissue diseases after receiving collagen injections even though they never had these diseases before. FDA is investigating whether there is a cause-and-effect relationship between having collagen treatments and later developing PM/DM or similar diseases.

Because collagen stays in the body and continues to be absorbed, the possible effects of collagen injections before or during pregnancy are unknown.

5) **Should doctors administering collagen injections provide patients with information on possible side effects of this product?** Yes. The manufacturers provide doctors with a patient brochure that explains the possible risks of collagen injections and identifies patients who should not receive this treatment. The package insert that doctors receive says that patients should be given a copy of this brochure before the final allergy test for collagen is performed.

6) **If a person is considering collagen injections, what should he or she discuss with the doctor?** In addition to reading the brochure carefully, patients should discuss with doctors the advantages and disadvantages of collagen injections, including how often treatments need to be repeated to maintain the effect. Patients should ask about the potential risks and tell the doctor about any history of allergies or connective tissue diseases such as rheumatoid arthritis or scleroderma.

LIQUID SILICONE INJECTIONS

1) **Has liquid silicone been approved by FDA for injection?** No. FDA has not approved the marketing of liquid silicone for injection for any cosmetic purpose, including the treatment of facial defects or wrinkles, or enlarging the breasts. The adverse effects of liquid silicone injections have included movement of the silicone to other parts of the body, inflammation and discoloration of surrounding tissues, and the formation of granulomas (nodules of granulated, inflamed tissue).

2) **Can FDA prohibit doctors from promoting the injection of liquid silicone, since its marketing has not been approved?** Yes. FDA prohibits manufacturers or doctors from marketing or promoting unapproved products such as liquid silicone. This means that the doctor cannot legally advertise or sell this material.

[Editor's note: A doctor can, however, inject liquid silicone if he feels that the patient would be best served by such an injection. The FDA's position is that they can only prohibit doctors and manufacturers from promoting, advertising, or selling this product because it is unapproved. They do not prohibit its use at the doctor's discretion. The law in California forbids silicone injections for breast augmentation only. Doctors may inject silicone legally in any other part of the body or face—KO]

COSMETIC SURGERY AND TEENS

INTRODUCTION

More and more teens are having cosmetic surgery to improve their looks. While we support reconstructive surgery for deformities or injuries, removal of unsightly birthmarks, etc., the authors of this book endorse no position on the pursuit of purely cosmetic, elective procedures by teenagers. This is a highly sensitive and controversial area.

The pro side is certainly persuasive. We have the technology to correct features which would otherwise subject a child to unmerciful teasing, or discomfort about his or her self-image (to which all teens, however stunning, fall prey), or problems with self-esteem. Why not save the young person from all that agony? Many parents feel, especially if it's an inherited feature, that they would prefer to spare their child the misery they went through themselves. It's a very good point—having self-confidence makes the humdrum battles in life easier to win, and also makes it easier to lose from time to time.

But should parents give their children the idea that looks are everything? Whatever happened to character, integrity, inner strength, the soul? Teens are not just growing physically;

they are developing skills and attitudes which will serve them as adults. Everyone must find their own balance for themselves, but parents have a responsibility to guide their children.

The decision to have cosmetic surgery requires a great deal of thought. The results are permanent. A teenager who has been thinking over a period of years about correcting a feature that bothers him or her is probably a good candidate. A child who wants his or her life to change dramatically after surgery is most likely not a good candidate. Parents and surgeons should plan on spending plenty of time with a teen discussing all of the feelings and options.

A teen might find after facial surgery that they have a great deal of trouble adjusting to their new face. I saw this recently in a teenage friend of mine. Prior to the surgery on her jaw, she was unable to close her mouth comfortably; she couldn't chew or even breathe or sleep normally, and her chin was farther back then it should have been. Her surgery wasn't purely for cosmetic reasons. After the surgery, she is most definitely prettier, although the change is so subtle that had I not known that she'd been through it, I would never have suspected that she'd had surgery. Yet her mother told me that she "hates" her face—the change is enormous to her; her face is suddenly not the face she has been looking at in the mirror for sixteen years. This is a reaction common to both teens and adults, and definitely needs to be addressed prior to surgery, especially surgery that's strictly for cosmetic reasons. You can't put your face back the way it was!

It's a good idea for a teen to think about cosmetic surgery for a long time. Give yourself a chance to grow into your body. If you're heavy, it's a healthier idea to establish an exercise program for yourself, and good eating habits—these will serve you well for your whole life, and contribute to your happiness now and as an adult. If your nose doesn't look right, I can tell you from personal experience that although your nose has matured by the time you're fifteen to seventeen years old, it might take until you're twenty-something for your body to catch up and your looks to balance out—naturally. And try the skillful use of cosmetics or hairstyles, too. Treat yourself to a really good cosmetic makeover and hair stylist, or ask for them as a birthday present. See what a difference it can make!

If a few years go by, and you're still really unhappy, that's the time to consult with a cosmetic or plastic surgeon. As a matter of fact, consult with several. You will be able to pick the right one for you by how comfortable he or she makes you feel, how thorough he or she is in answering your questions, how much time he or she spends with you—in addition to his/ her reputation and qualifications.

At the same time, consider what makes you happy. Think of your hobbies, your friends, your interests. Do you like yourself as a person? Are you a good friend? Would you choose yourself for a friend, looks aside? List to yourself all of the good personal qualities that you have. Praise yourself for your strengths, and make a deal with yourself to work on your weaknesses. And keep in mind that since nobody's perfect, you're as perfect as anyone can be just by being you!

EGGED ON BY MOMS, MANY TEEN-AGERS GET PLASTIC SURGERY

By Suzanne Alexander

Staff Reporter of the
The Wall Street Journal
September 24, 1990

As an eighth-grade graduation present, Kristina Olson got new ears from her mother. Leigh Kane, at 17, got a new nose.

Since last month, Danielle Borngiorno, 14, has had narrower hips and thinner thighs. Her mother offered to pay for breast implants, but Danielle decided against that, for the time being. She is still considering chin and nose work and a cheek implant. "Now, [it's] just like, let's go every week and get something improved on. There are so many things you can do," says Danielle, who lives in Brooklyn, N.Y.

Why bother with padded bras and Clearasil when silicone and dermabrasion promise permanence? Why spend one's adolescence brooding about receding chins or big ears when it is so simple to have plastic surgery?

To the dismay of at least some psychologists and medical doctors, cosmetic surgery is now hardly more exotic than orthodontics among children whose parents have the where-withal to pay $600 or $6,000 for a surgical procedure to improve on nature. Statistics don't exist, but many plastic surgeons say their teen-age clientele has doubled in the past five years and now is as much as 25% of their business.

Nose and ear jobs remain the most popular operations. But dermabrasion (sanding off layers of skin), breast augmentation and liposuction (fat sucking) are coming on strong with kids, not just with middle-aged entertainers like Phyllis Diller. Many Asian boys and girls, overeager to assimilate, seek to reshape the epicanthic fold in their eyelids. Some black youths, a la Michael Jackson, see surgeons for narrower noses and thinner lips.

Observers critical of the phenomenon see in it pampered children who can't tolerate the pain of being themselves. They see a society obsessed with appearance and with narrow-minded notions of what constitutes beauty.

"I hear doctors defend the right of teens to have face-lift surgery and eyelid surgery," says Frederick Stucker, chairman of the Otolaryngology-Head and Neck Surgery Department at Louisiana State University, "but I think we send the wrong message when we're willing to do it for teens." Dr. Stucker maintains that a lot of operations are unnecessary because teenage acne, babyfat and other "problems" usually disappear on their own as kids get older.

Adds Norman M. Cole, vice president of the American Society of Plastic and Reconstructive Surgeons: "A real problem in our society is that parents want everything for their children. Aesthetic surgery has become a commodity. 'I want my son to have a new stereo, car, nose and chin.' This is something that deserves some careful interrogation." Surgery to change racial characteristics, Dr. Cole says, is "an inappropriate concession to Western images. The Oriental eye in China is considered the most beautiful in the world. It's a sad commentary. . . . "

Cosmetic surgeons have their own interests in the matter, and some of them argue that plastic surgery is a real boon to teen-agers psychologically. Insecurity, self-consciousness and a lack of self-esteem vanish once the bandages come off. Surgery can take "years off a psychiatrist's couch," says Walter Berman, a facial plastic surgeon in Beverly Hills, Calif.

"I did two kids [a 14-year-old girl and a 16-year-old boy] this week who had a hereditary bagging of the upper eyelid," says Lori Hansen, a plastic surgeon in Oklahoma City, Okla. "It made them look tired all the time. So we just took the extra skin and fat away. Things are so easily fixed now. We don't have to live with them."

But critics say that in many cases parents are to blame for wanting "perfect-looking" children, thus encouraging low self-esteem in their offspring. "We see it often," says Pearlman D. Hicks, a plastic surgeon in Long Beach, Calif. "The parent tells the kid, 'Your nose looks terrible. You don't even look like part of the family.' [Parents] plant the seed and get the kids worried."

Nose jobs, of course, are nothing new for teen-agers. But they once were a thing of the affluent and the disfigured. Now, middle-class people get them almost willy-nilly. They are a socially acceptable mid-course correction in the life of an adolescent. New procedures, like liposuction, have been introduced in the U.S. within the past 10 years and pull in a lot of patients.

Many teen-agers who have had cosmetic surgery say they are glad they did. Why put it off and prolong the agony when they are likely to have it done eventually anyway?

Kristina Olson, 20, of Indianapolis, used to hate to go to school because her "Dumbo" ears, as she refers to them, stuck out. "I couldn't enjoy life," says Kristina, who would sit in the back of the classroom and hold her hand over one ear while covering the other with her hair.

Finally, her mother took her in for otoplasty—which, in effect, pins back protruding ears—as a gift of "happiness and mental health." At the age of 16, Kristina entered a new school and "no one knew the history of my ears." Her self-esteem and self-confidence soared.

One young black woman, who doesn't want her name mentioned, thought her nose was too wide. While she didn't want to change all her racial features, the 19-year old thought a smaller, narrower nose would "enhance" her beauty.

So, after white friends of hers had rhinoplasties done and her own father had the surgery, the Los Angeles resident, now 21, decided to narrow her nose, too. "I don't think I'm trying to be white," although she realizes that "a lot of people see it that way."

Leigh Kane, of Glen Cove, N.Y., the boy who had the nose job at 17, says he hadn't realized his nose was out of the ordinary until his mother told him so two years ago. "I thought she was kidding. [She said] she noticed that it was getting progressively worse as I got older," says Leigh, now 19. Suddenly self-conscious, Leigh had a surgeon remove a bump on his nose and fashion a new tip. And now he feels better about himself.

Despite the anecdotal evidence from satisfied young clients, medical professionals worry that youngsters aren't prepared to cope with the perils—physical and psychological—of cosmetic surgery.

"I think the psychological risk among teens is significantly higher than it is among [the] more mature," says Dr. Cole. Often teen-agers and their parents have unrealistic expectations that changing appearance will solve deep-seated problems that require psychiatric attention, not cosmetic surgery.

Dr. Cole says that several years ago he performed rhinoplasty on a 16-year-old-girl who was ecstatic with the results at first but later returned complaining that the nose job hadn't done the trick. She couldn't, however, articulate exactly what was bothering her, "I think psychologically . . . that nose wasn't the problem," he says.

Since most surgical procedures are irreversible, operating on teen-agers is a heavy responsibility. Patients are routinely told that things can't be put back the way they were after the surgery has been done. Patients are counseled extensively before surgery, so they know the risks involved. In most states, an 18-year-old can get plastic surgery without parental consent. Still, some young patients and their families have regrets.

Dr. Cole says a colleague operated on the eyelids of an 18-

year-old youngster of Korean ancestry who panicked because his grandparents were angry. "The family was insulted," Dr. Cole says. They felt that, in having the surgery, the young man was rejecting his culture. He went back in desperation seeking to have the surgery undone, but of course it wasn't possible.

Doctors say that to be unhappy with one's physical appearance is simply part of being a teen-ager, and that maturity can be the cure. Michael Seifert, 14, of Los Angeles, has a bump on his nose and a father who is a plastic surgeon. The son wanted surgery. The father refused on the grounds that Michael is too young.

Lately, Michael has found a new girl-friend, who thinks the bump on his nose gives him "character." He no longer wants to go under the knife.

FACIAL PLASTIC
SURGERY FOR TEENS
A PARENT'S GUIDE

The time to see a surgeon is when the child expresses serious concerns about a feature that may be corrected through facial plastic surgery. Don't pressure the child. The exceptions to this rule are if your child has protruding ears, a port wine stain, or other birth defects. Parents might encourage early consideration of correction for these problems to save their child a lifetime of teasing. Corrective procedures can be done effectively at a young age.

There is always benefit to learning how a problem will be affected by normal growth, and at what point surgical intervention might be helpful. An early consultation with a facial plastic surgeon will help you learn how to monitor growth and give you time to prepare for surgery if it is needed.

Protruding ears and some birth defects most frequently are corrected before a child starts school. If the child has a functional problem—such as an underdeveloped lower jaw—see the doctor early to determine what the appropriate course of treatment should be. Other procedures are not done until the face has reached its full growth. This is usually 14 or 15 years of

Reprinted by courtesy of The American Academy of Facial Plastic and Reconstructive Surgeons.

age for girls and 16 or 17 for boys.

Teens who are seeking perfection or who wish to look like someone else—say a movie star or a particular model—are not considered good candidates for facial plastic surgery. Most people who have surgery are well-adjusted individuals who basically like themselves but wish to change a feature with which they are dissatisfied.

The surgeon you consult will spend as much time as necessary to help you and your child make this decision. The child's emotional and physical well-being will be discussed as it relates to his or her being a good candidate for surgery.

Since healing differs with each individual, the surgeon cannot promise a specific result. However, facial plastic surgeons use several methods to show how a person's unique bone structure and covering tissues may react to surgery. These techniques—including sketching, use of mathematical measurements, and computer imaging—also may be used to demonstrate how a feature may change as the child matures.

It is important to choose a surgeon with whom you and your child feel comfortable and confident. You may want to get a referral from your family doctor or ask friends and relatives who have had facial plastic surgery. Try to find a doctor who relates to teenagers, who listens well and takes plenty of time to answer any questions you or your teenager might have.

Be sure to look for a facial plastic surgeon who specializes in the particular procedure your child wants and who consistently gets good results.

Facial plastic surgery cannot produce a miracle. Anyone who expects it to be the answer to personal problems is likely to be disappointed. Facial plastic surgery can minimize facial problems and improve appearance. The improvement, in turn, may enhance self-confidence. But surgery should not be expected to improve a teenager's social life or solve other problems.

The final results depend on the skill and experience of the

surgeon, as well as the age, health, skin texture, bone structure, and healing capacity of the patient. A positive emotional attitude also is important. Young patients generally heal quickly and experience good results.

TEENS DISCUSS FACIAL PLASTIC SURGERY

from *The Teen Face Book,*
prepared by the American Academy of Facial
Plastic and Reconstructive Surgeons

Tracey had always hated her nose. "I would never consider going out without makeup on," she recalls. "I did everything to try and cover it up, and I never let people see my profile. But the nose really defines the face, and when you have a nose like mine was, there is really no way to hide it."

No matter how she tried to disguise her nose, Tracey remained extremely self-conscious. "I was upset every time I looked in the mirror," she says. "My nose wasn't a deformity, exactly, but in my eyes it was very unattractive."

From the time she was 14, Tracey knew she would seek a permanent solution to her problem—facial plastic surgery. Although some teens may consider facial plastic surgery a rather drastic solution, for Tracey, who lives in suburban New York City, it was not unusual. "You have to understand that cosmetic surgery is very popular here. For girls between the ages of 14 and 20, having a rhinoplasty [nasal surgery] is not a rare thing." At first Tracey's parents didn't agree. They felt she looked just fine. "But they knew how I felt about my nose, and once they understood I was determined to have the surgery,

Reprinted by permission of the American Academy of Facial Plastic and Reconstructive Surgeons.

they supported me 100 percent." They all agreed she would wait until she was 17 to have the surgery.

Two years after her surgery, Tracey remains enthusiastic. "The biggest change has been in my personality. Before the surgery I was inhibited and shy because I always thought people were looking at my nose. Today I like the way I look, so I'm more outgoing." Tracey notes that she read a great deal about how to improve her appearance before deciding to have surgery. That is essential, she and other patients feel, to understanding exactly what can be accomplished with a cosmetic makeover or a new hairstyle—and what may be correctable only through facial plastic surgery.

Penny, 16, found the courage to audition for a slot on the cheerleading squad even though she was overweight and considered unattractive by her peers. She wasn't booed, exactly, but when the student body voted, Penny was at the bottom of the list.

"At our school, parking lot assignments were decided by the student body president, who was a guy," confides Terry, 16. "All the paved parking spaces went to the pretty girls and to his buddies."

Face it. In today's culture, looks do count, especially for teens. Whether it's a modeling job or just a date for the senior prom, your appearance is on the line. You may wish that society was less judgmental, but you have to accept that how you look affects how people relate to you—and often how you relate to them.

"Everyone knows that the good-looking guys don't date ugly girls or girls who are fat," points out Susan, age 15.

"Student Council and especially Homecoming Court—these people are always chosen for their looks, not their personality," comments Jennifer, 17.

"Often the teacher will walk into a class on the first day and decide by your looks how he will treat you for the entire year," maintains Sean, 16.

Many teens understandably are dismayed with this focus on

looks, even as they acknowledge it exists. "What in history has caused mankind to put so much emphasis on looks?" laments Joel, 17. "Whatever happened to inner beauty?" Another young man, age 16, comments, "People shouldn't be that concerned with their facial features. We shouldn't allow people to make us feel inferior because of them." "I always try my best to look good," says Sara, 14, "but I sure wish looks weren't that important."

. . . Nearly all know at least one friend or classmate who is not particularly attractive, but, because he or she has a classy personality or witty sense of humor, is a lot of fun to be with. These individuals have gone beyond their looks and have, as one teen bluntly remarked, "broken the ugly barrier."

"There are many unattractive people I like for their personality," acknowledges Dianna, 14. "A smile and a sense of humor go a long way in making friends."

Carey, 17, notes, "I know a girl who isn't pretty at all. She has a very crooked nose. People call her names and laugh, but she laughs right along with them. She has a great attitude toward life."

"The wittiest boy in our class is also the ugliest," notes David, 14. "I think he is very bold and courageous."

It also is true that "beauty is in the eye of the beholder." Often a person will worry about some detail of his or her appearance that others don't even notice. It's easy for a young person to begin worrying more and more about a facial "blemish" that actually is perfectly normal. Before you start worrying about your facial features, take a minute to look at others your age who are popular. Chances are, most of them don't have "perfect" features.

Looks that are too perfect can be a liability, too. Both guys and girls feel that the best looking of their classmates often let it go to their head. Such individuals are accused of acting stuck-up or snobbish.

"I'm really suspicious if a guy who is too good-looking asks me out," comments Karen, 19. "That intimidates me. I wonder why he's doing it."

"A friend of mine actually lost a job because she was too pretty," relates Susan, 15. "The boss didn't want a lot of guys hanging around."

At first glance, this emphasis on appearance seems superficial and vain, but on second analysis it may not be all bad.

The point to looking your best, says psychologist Dr. Joyce Brothers, is to be able to forget about yourself and be self-confident. "When you look good and feel great, people treat you as if you're special," she says. "Your appearance sends signals to others about who you are, how you feel, even about your values and aspirations. When people treat you as if you are intelligent and friendly, you behave that way, and that starts an upward spiral of success."

Other psychologists, too, regard a little vanity as a good thing. Attention to one's looks is a sign of self-esteem, just as lack of interest in grooming and appearance is an early sign of depression. Thus, appearance has a lot to do with how you feel about yourself, both inside and outside. It helps to shape your self-image.

"If I feel I look good in the morning, then I feel good all day long," points out Amy, 19, speaking for a lot of her peers.

"When I look at myself in the mirror, I see an average-looking person," says Marcy, 16. "If my acne is bad at the time or I just don't look my best, I tend to be in a bad mood or depressed about my looks. If I look good, I'm in a better mood and I feel good and self-confident about myself."

"I have a friend whose mood and self-confidence depend entirely on how his hair looks. If his hair was cut to the middle of his neck without his knowledge, it is safe to say his self-confidence would all but disappear and his mood would shift from arrogant to withdrawn and extremely shy," notes Marc, 19. It is no secret that young people spend a great deal of time working at looking good. And it's perfectly healthy and normal to try to make the best of your appearance.

As Lisa Sliwa, national director of the Guardian Angels,

noted in an interview in *Vogue* magazine, it's balance that counts. "To be obsessed with your appearance is unhealthy. But if you look at improving your physical appearance as part of your overall life strategy, it's empowering."

Complexion, hair, and eyes top the list of facial features that most concern guys and girls of all ages. But they have other concerns. Teens want to know how to make their lips look larger—and their noses smaller. They are worried about oily skin, ears that protrude, and the dangers of too much sun. Moles and birthmarks, plump cheeks, and weak chins also cause frustration.

Moreover, despite all of the literature on the subject, teens still aren't sure exactly how drugs, smoking, alcohol, diet, and exercise affect their appearance.

Cosmetics and skincare products expertly used can cover a multitude of facial imperfections. Healthful living, personality, and an inner glow count, too. But there is another option, especially for problems of a more structural nature, and that is facial plastic surgery. For teens in many parts of the country, facial plastic surgery as a cosmetic option is a very new idea.

Rachel, of suburban New York, has several friends who would never think of having cosmetic surgery, and she feels that's great, for them. "But it was the best thing I ever did in my life," she says of her nasal surgery five years ago when she was 13. "It saved me from a future of insecurities."

Toni, 16, who also had facial plastic surgery, acknowledges that focusing on appearance should not be that important. "But I had to be pretty before I could say that."

On the other hand, Jon, 15, says he would never consider surgery unless he was in a disfiguring accident. "We should accept the face we were born with," he maintains.

The point is that facial surgery is a very important personal decision. The degree of your facial problem isn't what's important, but how you feel about it is. If your looks bother you on a regular basis, if they are a source of embarrassment or present problems that you cannot address with cosmetics, hairstyle, or more conventional measures, then facial plastic surgery may be right for you. . . .

The danger is in believing that facial plastic surgery can change your life. It can't. In fact, the very best facial plastic surgery won't drastically change your looks unless your appearance is quite misshapen to begin with. "When I went to school people knew I looked better, but they didn't exactly know why" is the comment that young facial plastic surgery patients make over and over.

Facial plastic surgery is not for everyone. It won't help you do better in school, and it won't win you friends. In and of itself, it can't get you a boyfriend or girlfriend. But, in some cases, it can help you feel better about yourself, and it can bring out the beauty you feel is hidden inside. For some people, facial plastic surgery relieves worry about appearance so that they can get on with life without focusing obsessively on looks.

COSMETIC SURGERY UPDATE

By Elizabeth Karlsberg

Teen
January 1991

According to Dr. [Harvey] Zarem [of Santa Monica, California], a female's nose is pretty well developed at age 13 or 14, although in some cases it may take longer. ("For males, there tends to be continued growth until 15 or 16, so unless [the nose] is a major problem, it's probably better to wait," notes Dr. Zarem.

When you go in for a rhinoplasty consultation, the doctor will also look closely at your jaws and perhaps even your teeth. You may look at your face and only see that you have a prominent nose. The plastic surgeon may see that your nose looks even more prominent because you also have a recessed chin. Someone else may have an overgrowth of the jaw.

"When looking at her nose, a teenager should also look at her teeth and jaws," says Dr. Zarem. "It's worth pointing out because more often than not, the patient comes in focused on her nose and is totally taken aback when we start talking about her chin. The problem may be simple or complex, but often, a good orthodontic evaluation is warranted."

You might be envious of a girl with very large breasts—until you had to carry them around with you every day. "Big breasts are uncomfortable for a young girl both physically and emotionally," explains Dr. Zarem. "Big breasts call attention to the girl, and can be very awkward for her socially."

Large, heavy breasts can also cause health problems, such as neck and back pain, as well as rounded shoulders. Also, Dr. Zarem says it's not uncommon for a girl with large breasts to be overweight. "Now she's not the girl with the big breasts, but the fat girl," he explains. "She can deal with [being fat] more readily than being the girl with the big breasts."

Breast surgery, called mammoplasty, can be used to either reduce the size of the breasts or augment. But plastic surgeons, such as Dr. Zarem and Dr. [Gregory] Wingate [of Phoenix, Arizona], also see a lot of young women who have breasts that are asymmetrical—one breast is significantly smaller than the other.

"On the other hand," adds Dr. Zarem, "there are a number of girls who seek breast augmentation because they are just simply flat-chested."

"Cosmetic surgery," says Dr. Wingate, "isn't for everybody. Some people, because of their own philosophies of body image, would never make good plastic surgery candidates."

In other words, if you're going to feel guilty about changing the YOU you were born with, you're better off just the way you are.

"To me, the distinction between improving someone's self-esteem and fueling their vanity is a very fine line," says Dr. Zarem. "One person may not mind being small-breasted, whereas it's a real problem for someone else. So each of us has our own individual perception of what's appropriate."

If you feel that your face or figure is among the fairest of them all, hats off to you! But, if your features don't quite seem to fit, and are causing you lots of frustration and heartache, fret not: Plastic surgery can help! The old cliché about beauty being in the eye of the beholder really does hold true. So, try to remember that what appears "flawed" to you, someone else just might fancy!

COMMON PROCEDURES FOR TEENAGERS

AAFPRS Backgrounder

Rhinoplasty — a procedure which improves the size and shape of the nose to bring it into harmony with the rest of the face. It is done by removing excess bone and cartilage and sculpting the remaining structures. Breathing problems may be corrected in a combined procedure called septorhinoplasty.

Mentoplasty [or genioplasty] (chin augmentation) — a procedure which helps correct a receding chin through insertion of a small plastic implant. Mentoplasties are often done in conjunction with nasal plastic surgery, and may be combined with liposuction or lipectomy procedures removing excess fat from beneath the chin.

Otoplasty — a procedure for "pinning back" protruding ears or correcting ear deformities.

Dermabrasion — a facial sanding procedure that is used to diminish severe acne and other scars.

Blepharoplasty — a procedure which is performed on young people who have unusually droopy, closed, or angry-looking eyes.

Courtesy of American Academy of Facial Plastic and Reconstructive Surgery.

BAD HABITS TO AVOID IF YOU VALUE YOUR APPEARANCE

from *The Teen Face Book*

There are all sorts of reasons to avoid smoking, drinking, and drugs— three life-threatening habits that teens are particularly susceptible to. One reason is appearance. Just as with the foods you eat, the toxins that you take into your body eventually will show up on your face. Let's looks at the damage they do.

SMOKING

- Constricts the small blood vessels of your face, reducing the supply of oxygen to delicate facial tissues. Eventually this will destroy that healthy glow that most teens admire, leaving you with a grayish "smoker's face."
- Contributes to lines around your face and eyes. Taking a drag on a cigarette causes your mouth to "purse up." While the lines may not be noticeable in the teen years, eventually the lines around your mouth become permanent. Wrinkles around your eyes develop even sooner— experts aren't sure if this is the result of reduced oxygen to your face or because cigarette smoke causes squinting.
- Stains your teeth and spoils your smile. Smoking also is

Courtesy of American Academy of Facial Plastic and Reconstructive Surgery.

directly linked to mouth and throat cancers. Incidentally, the chewing tobacco popular today might not make your clothes smell bad, but it does stain your teeth and contribute to oral cancer.

DRUGS

- Cause acne flare-up [especially "speed" or amphetamines].
- Suppress circulation to your skin, causing it to lose its natural color and look gray and tired. This is true of both stimulants and depressants, including the caffeine that is in colas, tea, and coffee.
- Contribute to nasal problems. This is a particular danger with cocaine, which can lead to nosebleeds and breathing difficulties, destroy the cartilage within your nose, and even cause your entire nose to collapse.
- Cause facial lines and wrinkles. This is as true of marijuana as it is of regular cigarettes.
- Cause fluid retention that results in a roundness or distortion of your face if the drugs are steroids or synthetic male hormones.

DRINKING

- Dehydrates your skin by drawing water away from its surface. Healthy skin needs this moisture.
- Increases the problem of broken capillaries.
- Causes blood vessels to expand, or dilate, increasing the redness of your skin. An alcohol "glow" is too red to look healthy.
- Lowers your physical reaction time, thus contributing to accidents, especially those involving motorcycles and automobiles. The facial damage from such accidents is a leading cause of facial disfigurement for teens.

EAT YOUR WAY TO GOOD LOOKS

Your Problem	What You Need	Where to Get It
Acne, skin eruptions, blotchy complexion	Vitamin A	Apricots, broccoli, milk, butter, spinach, tangerines.
	Zinc	Liver, dark turkey meat, whole-grain breads, bran.
	Vitamins B-1, B-2, and B-6	Meat, Fish, poultry, whole-grain breads and cereals, many fruits and vegetables.
Flabby skin	Silenium maintains the skin's elasticity; too much, though, can be toxic.	Poultry, seafood, red meat.
Pale complexion	Folic acid	Asparagus, broccoli, spinach, liver.
Bleeding gums	Vitamin C	Citrus fruits, cantaloupe, berries, tomatoes, broccoli.
Tooth decay	Calcium	Skim milk, cheese, yogurt.
	Vitamin D	Fortified milk, liver, eggs, fish.
Dull, lifeless hair	Vitamin B-12	Lean meat, fish, eggs, milk, liver.
Premature hair loss	Zinc	Liver, dark turkey meat, whole-grain breads, bran.

From *The Teen Face Book*, © 1989. Courtesy of American Academy of Facial Plastic and Reconstructive Surgery.

WORST-CASE
SCENARIOS

INTRODUCTION

Most cosmetic surgery procedures succeed in their purpose. The patient might be sore and bruised, might take a while to get used to a new physical feature, might have secretly wished for more spectacular results in the rest of his or her life. For the most part, however, everyone is happy—the patient with the result and the doctor with the satisfaction of a job well done (and well paid).

Sometimes things are not so rosy. Any procedure can go very wrong. The following are true stories from court and congressional documents which illustrate *how* wrong. Some of the surgeons represented here are highly renowned and respected, and some have since lost their licenses for malpractice. Some are "cosmetics" and some are "plastics." Some made honest mistakes, and some were inexcusably careless or cavalier.

How can a cosmetic surgery candidate avoid such trouble? Know your surgeon, know every aspect of the procedure, and keep your fingers crossed.

CONGRESSIONAL TESTIMONY

STATEMENT OF JOYCE P

Before the Subcommittee on Regulation,
Business Opportunities & Energy
April 4, 1989

Five years ago, I was a very happy, very healthy middle aged woman who owned a prosperous business that was growing by leaps and bounds. I began to notice so many advertisements about cosmetic surgery—it all sounded so simple. I decided I could stand a tuck here and there to improve my looks and perhaps look younger. The ads almost sounded like going to get a tooth filled—go in in the morning, have a tummy tuck done, a face lift, or a breast enlargement and go home in the afternoon. No need to go to a hospital—doctors were doing these procedures in their offices.

I thought this must be safe, or who in the medical profession or government would allow doctors to do this? I thought things like that were controlled by the AMA., the states or at least someone. So I went for consultations with five plastic surgeons. Several could not schedule me in when I needed because of my work schedule. I found one close to my home who could fit me in. I talked about a tummy tuck, a breast lift and a face lift at the same time.

I asked for a list of his credentials and for names of patients whom he had done these procedures on. His list of credentials looked quite impressive. I know now that most of the things he had listed meant absolutely nothing other than the fact that he did have an M.D. degree. I called AMA. in Chicago to check on him. I was told that he "was a member in good standing." I now know what that meant was only that he had paid his dues. I called the California Board of Medical Quality Assurance in Sacramento and asked about this doctor. They told me "they had nothing on him." I thought that meant they had nothing negative on him. He also had listed University of California, Davis. I called them and was told that he may have attended a seminar there regarding plastic surgery. The person on the line then told me to be sure I chose a Board Certified Surgeon. I looked on the doctor's credentials and noticed he had listed that he was a member of the Board of Cosmetic Surgeons.

. . .

From what I had been told and from his very impressive credentials that he had given me, I then asked to talk with some of his patients. I did meet with and talk with three of them. I believe, but I cannot be sure, that two of the three were decoys.

. . .

I went into his office very early on the morning of August 27, 1984. He performed a tummy tuck on me. That surgery requires a 12" incision from hip bone to hip bone. I went home at 4:00 that afternoon. Then I went back to his office the next Wednesday for him to remove drains. Then I went again on Friday. He told me not to change the bandage or look at the incision. I should have thought that was strange also, but I didn't question it at the time. The next Monday was a holiday so I did not go back until the next Wednesday—five days after the last visit when he told me not to change the bandage.

On the 9th day, he began to remove the sutures and said that something was not right, but, "not to worry, everything would be okay." I had been coughing and complained of the coughing. He said it was just the after-effects of surgery.

On the 10th day after surgery, I noticed seeping coming through the bandage. I took the bandage off and saw something very frightening. It looked like two coal black places, each the size of a tablespoon and another red, bloody, pussy place the same size. I called his office and was told that he was not in, to put another bandage on and come in the next day.

Shortly after that, he told me there was some infection, but that it would be okay. The wound then began to have a terrible odor, I was still coughing and had become short of breath all of the time. Each time that I would go in, I would tell him the same complaints—he kept saying it was the after-effects of surgery. He changed antibiotics three times.

Finally, at my suggestion, he took a culture and I heard him talk to the lab about the report. Apparently, they told him that those particular infections (there were three different kinds) never respond to oral antibiotics. He said he did not want to give injectibles. When I asked him why, he said that it would be expensive for me. I remember saying that I did not care—I just wanted to get well.

By this time, I was getting very weak and was very short of breath. Against his advice, I went for another opinion the very next day after I last saw him. When I . . . told another doctor what was happening, he told me to get a chest x-ray before I even came to his office. The doctor that performed the tummy tuck—even with all my complaints—had *never* taken my blood pressure, a blood test, listened to my heart or suggested a chest x-ray.

By the time I reached the other doctor's office, he had the x-ray, looked at the open, gaping wound, and called a pulmonary specialist. He told my daughter, who had taken me in to the office, to get me to the emergency room at the hospital immediately. The pulmonary specialist was there when I got there. They thought I had blood clots in my lungs. After many tests, lung scans, etc., the pulmonary specialist extracted a cup of fluid from my left lung. Also in the emergency room, they started cleaning out the wound. I looked and saw what looked like a crater full of blood and greenish looking pudding. . . . In a *very* short time, five different specialists [were] on my case. The pulmonary specialist discovered that there was something wrong with my heart and called in a cardiologist.

After the tests, it was discovered that the infection from the wound had gotten into my blood stream and had landed on the mitral valve in my heart. An infectious disease specialist was called in, an internist, and another "real" plastic surgeon. After being in the emergency room for seven hours, I was admitted as an inpatient.

The cardiologist came into my room the next day and explained to me what had happened. He told me that I had saved my own life by getting a second opinion when I did. If I had waited much longer, I would not be here today to tell this story.

He told me that the mitral valve was so damaged by the infections that I would have to undergo open heart surgery, but that they could not operate until the infection was under control. The infections were staph, pseudemonous and one other which they began to treat with intravenous antibiotics—two different ones. The wound was cleaned every three hours. I was in the hospital for two weeks, had some health care for four weeks, was taught to infuse my own antibiotics through a heparin lock, and had to go back to the hospital for six weeks for hydrotherapy and cleaning of the wound.

In one year I was in and out of the hospital six times. I also went into heart failure five times. The infections would not go away, so my doctors decided to open me up to see if they could find out the reason. *But* because of my heart, they could not give me general anesthetic, so I was awake under local anesthetic when they opened me up. They found a foot of suture that the doctor had left inside me and the infection was clinging to that suture.

After that, the infections would go away, then they would pop up again. We had the heart surgery scheduled for August, 1985, but then the infections appeared again so it had to be postponed.

Six days before Christmas in 1985, I had a stroke. The defective valve threw a clot which landed in the right side of my brain, affecting my left side. I could not talk and I could not swallow. Heart surgery was scheduled for February 11, 1986.

When I was rolled into surgery, I did not know if I would ever see my children again. Thanks to all my doctors who saved my life, I am now, four and a half years later, living a normal life. I must listen to the tick of my artificial mechanical valve in my heart. I hear it tick with every heart beat. I am on blood thinner for the rest of my life, so I must be very careful not to cut myself or I could lose a dangerous amount of blood. I must live with the horrible scars on my abdomen because my doctors will not allow me to have reconstructive surgery. I must go to the doctor once a month for life.

Needless to say, I lost all my business when this happened to me. Today, I am in the process of trying to rebuild that business. I lost a large amount of money which I will never be able to recoup. But I want to tell you this: *IT IS GREAT TO BE ALIVE.* The doctor who did the tummy tuck on me did the same procedure on a 36-year old registered nurse two months after he did me. She died from the same complications and infections that I had. *SO I AM THE LUCKY ONE.*

. . . no one has any control—as long as a person has an MD degree he can advertise and do anything he wants to do, anywhere he wants to do it. When the California State Investigator came to see me, she told me that they had been trying to get the doctor's license away for two years before I went to him, and that he had eleven lawsuits against him when I went to him. I asked why, when I called Sacramento, they had not told me that. She said that he had not been proven guilty on any of the cases so they couldn't tell me. It takes sometimes four and one half years to get a trial date for medical malpractice in California, so does that mean in the meantime that these guys can keep cutting on people? In my case, it did.

It took my case and the woman who died to get his license

revoked . . .

The AMA has no control. DO THEY CARE? The State Medical Quality Assurance Boards have their hands tied by the judicial system and a backlog of so many cases and a shortage of staff. The federal government apparently has no control.

. . .

Some of these doctors are very clever and can form whatever board they want to, get a group together, pay some kind of dues, go to a local printer and have impressive certificates made up to hang on their walls. DOES THAT QUALIFY THESE DOCTORS TO DO WHAT THEY ARE DOING? Does attending a seminar or course qualify these doctors to do what they are doing? I AM LIVING PROOF THAT IT DOES NOT!

. . .

Shouldn't the government, at the very least, stop doctors' ads that lull us into a false sense of security? Shouldn't ads that make us believe that we can have cosmetic surgery done safely and well with *no* risk be stopped?

CONGRESSIONAL
TESTIMONY

STATEMENT OF ANGELA B.

Before the Subcommittee on Regulation,
Business Opportunities & Energy
April 4, 1989

My name is Angela B. Before I tell you what happened to me, I want to express my gratitude that you are trying to educate the public about the seriousness of liposuction.

I chose to have liposurgery only after years of exercise and dieting that did not remove the saddlebags—that excess fat on the sides of my thighs.

I was led to believe that liposurgery was simple and successful. And since I felt that I had chosen a qualified board-certified plastic and reconstructive surgeon, I was sure everything would be just fine.

When I had a preliminary conference with the doctor, he told me, "You have good skin tone. You're not overweight, and the results will be great." I underwent surgery on May 13, 1987. Little did I know that after the surgery I would never be the same: not just in my outward appearance, but in my mental and emotional state, as well. I was in surgery for over two hours, as opposed to the initial 45 minutes the doctor said it would take to remove my saddlebags. This was due to the lipo machine which kept breaking down.

After the operation, I felt fine. I asked the nurse how much fat was removed. She replied, "lots more than I thought you had." She showed me a jar filled with my yellow fat. It looked like chicken grease.

Shortly afterwards, I went home and felt fine. About three or four weeks after the surgery I noticed my right leg was caving in and was sensitive to the touch. So, I called the doctor and went for a check-up. As soon as he saw it, he calmly said,

"I took out too much fat."

"Can it be corrected?" I asked.

"Yes, if it does not fill in, we can do fat grafts. That is when we remove fat from other areas of your body and use it to fill in and plump up the leg, but don't worry. You won't need it. Just rub your leg. Get your husband to massage it. Just think of all those good rub downs," he said with a snide grin.

However, my leg got worse. An area six inches long and six inches wide ran down the front of my right thigh. I could place my whole hand in the area. I could feel the muscle and the bone in my leg. The area was rock hard and it hurt.

Also, the skin tone was different. After a warm bath or shower the area would turn dark purple. My knee became three times its normal size. I could not bend my leg, nor put any pressure on it. I again returned to the doctor. Once more he told me, "Don't worry. Scar tissue is making the leg hard. Gradually the knee will return to normal. It's swollen due to the pressure of the scar tissue in your leg."

I kept returning to the doctor for months. Every visit with him was exactly like the previous one. I finally had to admit that my leg would not correct itself. Therefore, I visited several doctors to get their opinions.

One prominent board-certified surgeon—another plastic surgeon—told me too much fat had been removed, and I'd need two or three operations. Even then he said he was not sure if it would be all right. Then, he launched into the dangers of liposurgery: infection, hemorrhaging, or even death. He wanted me to sign a prepared paper stating everything that could go wrong, so if it did, he could not be sued for malpractice. I refused and visited another doctor.

As I entered this board-certified doctor's office, I saw a big sign: "Treat yourself to a tummy tuck on your VISA Card and a buttock lift on your MASTERCARD." I was shocked. I had never heard of this before.

This doctor told me the same story. I had a 50-50 chance of having it corrected in three operations, *costing $25,000*. He was supposed to be the best doctor, but after I overheard him quote a $6,500 fee for surgery to one woman and then cut it in half to $3,500 because she had a prior surgery with him, I felt irate. He was charging me an exorbitant fee—out of line with the cut-rate fee he was charging her.

So, I paid the fee for his consultation and left—still an unhappy woman.

Then while watching television, I saw an advertisement for the Cosmetic Surgery Center. I figured, I've been damaged by one board-certified surgeon and visited two other board-certified physicians, who appeared to be money-grubbing specialists, so I had nothing to lose by seeing what this other option could be.

At the Center, I was introduced to Dr. Antonio Mangubat. He told me he had performed over 1,200 liposurgeries. Even though he was not board-certified, I trusted his record. He explained his procedure to me. Because liposurgery is an art dependent on experience as well as knowledge, his success record meant a great deal to me.

The difference between the initial board-certified doctor who ruined my leg and Dr. Mangubat who corrected it was astronomical. Dr. Mangubat gave me hope. He was truly concerned and genuinely wanted to help me—not just for the money.

Dr. Mangubat took a long time talking with me. He measured my leg and the other parts of my body from which he would remove fat. He and his nurse took numerous pictures of me. Then Dr. Mangubat wrote the prescriptions in advance for the antibiotics and pain pills I would need after the operation when I went home.

Even though I was quite nervous, Dr. Mangubat and his staff made me feel comfortable. Before the surgery, Dr. Mangubat took more photographs. Then, he marked up the parts of my body from where the fat would be removed with a green magic marker. He practiced careful medicine, taking blood tests and being scrupulously careful about sterile instruments and the dangers of infection. These were things the original doctor did not do.

After the sedation took effect, the doctor used his liposuction machine to remove fat from my left leg (which I had not realized was three inches larger than my right leg in the upper back of the thighs). This evened out the dents that were there. More fat was removed from my stomach and upper arms. This filled in the cavity.

I knew I had to wait three weeks to see if the fat cells would take. Since 50 percent of the fat cells are supposed to die, I hoped that the doctor had inserted sufficient fat.

After the operation my right leg was severely swollen and hurt with a throbbing intensity.

I realized then that undergoing surgery to become slim and trim was not an issue to be considered trivially. Liposurgery is surgery. Things can and do go wrong.

Many people have admitted to me that they too have had problems. Yet, they felt ashamed to admit that the elective operation did not come out correctly. Many of the men and women who have undergone liposurgery need corrective operations but are either afraid or too ashamed to have them.

They suffer silently.

I will not be silent about the dangers of liposurgery. I am very pleased that this Committee has chosen to expose the problem and help the thousands of people who are unaware of the problems inherent in liposurgery, or of the unscrupulous and unskilled doctors who may be board-certified surgeons but still be butchers and calculating money makers.

Yes, I am ok now—except for a small fat pocket on my leg, and eventually I'll have this removed. But I would warn people to carefully consider whether the extra perfection is worth the risk.

COURT RECORDS

THE CASE OF MARVIS F.

On or about November 16, 1984, respondent performed an abdominoplasty and lipolysis on this patient in his medical office. The patient weighed 160 pounds and suffered from [a high white-blood cell count, indicative of an infection]. The patient went home after surgery, with instruction that she was to remain in a bent position, with no stress placed on her abdomen. On November 18, the patient's vital signs were high, and she was pale and [clammy]. Respondent gave her instructions by telephone that the top of her binders be loosened, and her pain medication be doubled. Marvis F. went to respondent's office on November 19, 21, and 23 to have the staples removed and the dressing changed. She did not see respondent.

On or about November 26, the suture line began to separate into a triangular shape. By December 2, the separation was 11 centimeters in height and 14 cm. in length. Fat and muscle became visible, and the wound began draining a thick, yellow, foul-smelling mucus. Marvis F. called respondent's office on November 26 to advise of this. A nurse told her that this was normal, to expect it, and to get some Kotex pads to use as dressings. Thereafter, until December 5, the dressing was changed every few hours by the patient or a friend. There was also considerable ecchymosis [the escape of blood into the tissues from ruptured blood vessels].

Respondent saw Marvis F. on November 30, by which time the wound was draining a yellow, purulent, foul-smelling discharge. Respondent performed a debridement [surgical removal of contaminated tissue] and took a culture. On December 3, 1984, respondent performed more debridement and placed her on ampicillin. By December 5, the wound was infected, there were extensive areas of abdominal wall necrosis [dead flesh] and the umbilicus could not be identified.

On December 5, Marvis F. went to Dr. Malcolm Paul who hospitalized her and on December 6 performed extensive debridement of the abdominal wall wounds with reconstruction. On December 14, she went home and was treated as an outpatient. On January 7, she was again hospitalized and [had the dead flesh from the remaining wounds cut away, necessitating skin grafts and further sutures to close the higher wounds]. Eventually, she went into shock and sustained a cardiac arrest. She died on January 17 of multiple pulmonary emboli.

COURT RECORDS

THE CASE OF JACKIE S.

On or about June 4, 1984, respondent performed a bilateral reduction mammoplasty on this patient in his medical office. Respondent did not send breast tissue to a pathologist. Shortly after surgery, she experienced excruciating pain on her left side between her breast, and over time, the pain worsened and expanded into her back, side, and chest cavity. The sutures began coming out and her left nipple turned black. Respondent told her there was dead skin which would slough off, and she would be all right . . . While the patient's right breast healed, the left breast drained and was painful. On June 28, respondent removed necrotic [dead] tissue from her left breast, performed debridement on June 29, July 2, and July 6, placed sutures in her left breast on July 6, and took a culture and gave her an injection on July 9. By July 11, the patient's wound was infected and there was an obvious loss of tissue of the skin and breast in the inferior portion of the left breast.

The patient went to another doctor on July 11. [Her] left breast requires reconstruction . . . to match her right breast, and scar removal.

COURT RECORDS

THE CASE SHARON B.

On January 8, 1982, respondent performed a facial chemical peel on Sharon B. During the procedure, the patient suffered cardiac arrythmia, was taken to an emergency room and then admitted to [the hospital]. She was discharged from the hospital on January 15 with a final diagnosis of hypoxic encephalopathy [lack of oxygen to the brain], improved, and chemical bronchitis secondary to ether inhalation.

Respondent's office note of [this] procedure contains the entry: "Ether kicked over by assistant. Pt began having cardiac arrythmia."

COURT RECORDS

THE CASE OF MELODY D.

On or about April 13, 1984, respondent performed a mammary augmentation by peri-areolar approach [incision around the areola] on Melody D. The patient was re-operated on in early May.

On May 14, Melody D.'s incision on her left breast opened, the implant protruded, and blood and fluid began oozing. The patient called respondent's office several times and left messages. Respondent did not call the patient back. Respondent's wife called Melody D. on May 15 and told the patient not to go to an emergency room.

On May 18, respondent removed the implant from the patient's left breast.

COURT RECORDS

THE CASE OF L.F.

L. F. heard about respondent on a Santa Ana radio station and went to see him for an abdominoplasty (tummy tuck). Respondent examined her and said he could remove all the excess skin; that she would still have a few stretch marks but that all the flabby skin would be removed. One of the females at the clinic took blood. The day of the operation, Ron M., unlicensed technician, injected her with Demerol. He also tried to get an I.V. started but could not find the vein. Leonard C. switched the I.V. to the other arm and started it.

L.F. remained while respondent operated on someone else. She was then taken into the "operating room." Respondent marked where he was going to cut, and then L.F. felt him start cutting and told him that it hurt. He told someone to put her under. The surgery took place. Afterward L. F. remained overnight in the office. The next day they had her walk a couple of times and she went home that evening. There she started running a fever and went back to the office. She was taking Tylenol and ampicillin for pain and infection. The incision was taped and it started oozing. Six days after the operation she again returned and respondent removed the tape—L. F.'s right side was split open! There was about a 1/2-inch deep gap open about 1/2 - 3/4 inches and about two inches long at the biggest part, and the rest of the cut was puckered.

Respondent said that he would not sew it up because it had to drain. Respondent had never shaved the area, and after the surgery, L. F. could pull hair out of the cut and a little pus would come out also.

About six weeks after the operation L. F. went back for a checkup. The side was healed but the scar was still very red. Respondent, who had taken pre-operation pictures, now took about 15 - 20 "after" shots, but he put makeup on the scar so it wouldn't be as noticeable.

COURT RECORDS

THE CASE OF KATHLEEN K.

On May 12, 1982, I had the complete facelift including an upper and lower lid blepharoplasty. . . . Following the surgery I had the normal bruising and swelling. Immediately following the surgery, the *inside* of my lower left eyelid was visible. In my ignorance, I had the idea that this condition would get better when the swelling and bruising subsided. After I had healed, my lower left eyelid still displayed the pink inside. The lower eyelids on both eyes sagged and the left, from the first, has been the most severe of the two. Both eyes were dry, red and irritated and always tearing.

I questioned Dr. G. and he told me if there was not some sag, that was a sign that not enough skin had been removed. Dr. G also told me that his very own lower eyelids were in that condition for two years after he had *his* facelift. I then told Dr. G. that I had not counted on two years of living with odd-shaped eyes.

In October, Dr. G . . . decided to do . . . something to repair the "pull" on the lower eyelids. On the [consent form] which I signed . . . the term is "Bilateral revision work on both lids to correct the pull." This consent did not inform me (nor did Dr. G.) that I would be left with a "Z" scar on the outer corners of both eyes. The left eye still sagged . . . even after this second surgery.

I feel completely foolish . . . How could I go from one procedure to another . . . with Dr. G. and still believe him? My ignorance of plastic surgery procedures and trust in Dr. G.'s recommendations is my only explanation . . . I was still not aware . . . that my problem was . . . that Dr. G. had removed *too much* from the lower eyelids.

My last surgery at Dr. G.'s hands was in July, 1983. This time . . . he would make an incision on the top of my head and work on the [eye] muscles from there. He did NOT inform me that he intended to remove part of my scalp. . . . My hairline is [now] an embarrassment I will live with for the rest of my life. When Dr. G. removed the bandages a day or two after this surgery I was aghast! I said, "Oh my God, I'm bald!' Dr. G. told me when my scalp softened and the stitches were removed, my hairline would drop a good bit. . . . As time progressed, I saw less and less of Dr. G., and when I did see him, he became less and less friendly and more defensive about my condition. . . .

I now have eye irritation. My husband tells me that my eyes do not close when I sleep . . . since the forehead lift, which also resulted in my raised hairline and loss of hair. . . . My professional background was with Hallmark Greeting Cards as a colorplate artist and designer. I find it much more difficult to paint . . . with my eye condition because I can only tolerate . . . fumes for very limited lengths of time. . . .

I retained an attorney. This attorney told me I would most probably have to go out of the area to find a qualified surgeon to testify against Dr. G. This was because Dr. G. was very powerful and no other physicians would cross him in his own area. . . . After approximately four months I received a letter from the attorney's secretary. She said the doctor to whom they had hope to refer me said *Dr. G.'s reputation is impeccable, above reproach.* . . . I could not find a single board-certified plastic surgeon to help me. The attorney promptly dropped my case.

I have seen five board-certified plastic surgeons and paid for consultations. Without exception, each said my hairline and hair condition is irretrievable. Four of the five said my eyes should be repaired, more for health reasons than cosmetic. All five refused to testify against Dr. G., even though three of the five said I certainly had grounds for a lawsuit. All five said they could not understand why he used the third procedure—removing the scalp—to work on the *lower* eyelids. Obviously, they all feared Dr. G. professionally and were unwilling to help me.

APPENDICES

APPENDICES

PHONE REFERENCE LIST

Aegis Analytical Laboratories, Inc.	(615) 331-5300
American Academy of Cosmetic Surgery	(312) 527-6713
Toll-Free	(800) 221-9808
American Academy of Facial Plastic and Reconstructive Surgery	(202) 842-4500
American Board of Medical Specialties	(312) 464-5000
American Board of Plastic Surgery	(215) 587-9322
American Medical Association	(312) 464-5000
American Society for Aesthetic Plastic Surgery	(708) 228-9274
Toll-Free	(800) 635-0635
American Society of Plastic and Reconstructive Surgeons, Inc.	(708) 228-9900
Toll-Free	(800) 635-0635
Command Trust Network	(606) 331-0055
Dow Corning Wright Breast Implant Hotline	
Patients	(800) 442-5442
Physicians	(800) 437-7056
Food and Drug Administration (FDA)	(301) 443-1544
FDA Breast Implant Information Hotline	(800) 532-4440

Federal Trade Commission (FTC)   (202) 326-2222

Federal Information Center
    For referrals to your local state agenices such as
    medical boards and questions about legislation
    or governing bodies, etc.   (800) 726-4995

Public Citizen Health Research Group   (202) 833-3000

AMERICAN BOARD OF MEDICAL SPECIALTIES

MEMBERS

American Board of Allergy & Immunology
American Board of Anesthesiology
American Board of Colon & Rectal Surgery
American Board of Dermatology
American Board of Emergency Medicine
American Board of Family Practice
American Board of Internal Medicine
American Board of Neurological Surgery
American Board of Nuclear Medicine
American Board of Obstetrics & Gynecology
American Board of Ophthalmology
American Board of Orthopaedic Surgery
American Board of Otolaryngology
American Board of Pathology
American Board of Pediatrics
American Board of Physical Medicine and Rehabilitation
American Board of Plastic Surgery
American Board of Preventive Medicine
American Board of Psychiatry & Neurology
American Board of Radiology
American Board of Surgery
American Board of Thoracic Surgery
American Board of Urology

SELF-DESIGNATED BOARDS

Information exists in the ABMS files on the following self-designated boards. They are called "American Board of _____" unless otherwise designated, and each purports to certify physicians.

Abdominal Surgeons
Acupuncture Medicine
Addictionology
Aesthetic Plastic Surgery
Alcoholism & Other Drug Dependencies (AMSAODD)
Algology (Chronic Pain)
Ambulatory Anesthesia
Anthroscopy
Arthroscopic Surgery

Courtesy of the American Board of Medical Specialties.

Bariatric Medicine
Bionic Medicine
Bloodless Medicine & Surgery
Cardiac Catheterization and Angiography
Chelation Therapy
Chemical Dependence
Clinical Chemistry
Clinical Ecology
Clinical Neurology
Clinical Neurophysiology
Clinical Nutrition
Clinical Orthopaedic Surgery
Clinical Pharmacology
Clinical Polysomnography
Clinical Psychiatry
Clinical Psychology
Clinical Toxicology
Cosmetic Plastic Surgery
Cosmetic Surgery
Council of Non-Board Certified Physicians
Critical Care in Medicine & Surgery
Disability Evaluating Physicians
Electrodiagnostic Medicine
Electroencephalography
Electromyography and Electrodiagnosis
Environmental Medicine
Epidemiology (College)
Facial Cosmetic Surgery
Facial Plastic Surgery
Forensic Psychiatry
Forensic Toxicology
Hand Surgery
Head, Facial & Neck Pain & TMJ Orthopedics
Health Physics
Homeotherapeutics
Hypnotic Anesthesiology, National Board for
Industrial Medicine & Surgery
Insurance Medicine
Int'l. Cosmetic & Plastic Facial Reconstr. Stds.
Interventional Radiology
Laser Surgery
Law in Medicine
Malpractice Physicians
Maxillofacial Surgeons
Medical Accreditation (American Federation for)
Medical Genetics
Medical Hypnosis

Medical Laboratory Immunology
Medical-Legal Analysis of Medicine & Surgery
Medical Legal & Workers Compensation Medicine & Surgery
Medical Legal Consultants
Medical Microbiology
Medical Preventics (Academy)
Medical Toxicology
Medical Psychotherapists
Microbiology (Medical Microbiology)
Military Medicine
Neurologic & Orthopaedic Dental Medicine & Surgery
Neurological & Orthopaedic Medicine
Neurological & Orthopaedic Surgery
Neurological Microsurgery
Neuro-Orthop. Dental Medicine & Surgery
Neuro-Orthop. Electrodiagnosis
Neuro-Orthop. Laser Surgery
Neuro-Orthop. Psychiatry
Neuro-Orthop. Thor. Medicine/Surgery
Nutrition
Orthopaedic Microneurosurgery
Otorhinolaryngology
Pain Management (American Academy of)
Pain Management Specialties
Pain Medicine
Percutaneous Diskectomy
Plastic Esthetic Surgeons
Prison Medicine
Psychiatric Medicine
Psychiatry (American National Board of)
Psychoanalysis (American Examining Board in)
Psychological Medicine (International)
Quality Assurance and Utilization Review
Radiology and Medical Imaging
Rheumatologic and Reconstructive Medicine
Ringside Medicine & Surgery
Skin Specialists
Spinal Cord Injury
Spinal Surgery
Sports Medicine/Surgery
Toxicology
Trauma Surgery
Traumatologic Medicine & Surgery
Tropical Medicine
Ultrasound Technology
Urologic Allied Health Professionals

TREATMENT LOCATIONS AND SURGEON'S FEES FOR 1990 ASPRS COSMETIC PATIENTS

PROCEDURE	SURGEON'S FEES*			TREATMENT LOCATION	
	LOW	HIGH	AVG.	INPATIENT	OUTPATIENT
Arm Lift	$1,000	$6,500	$2,210	47%	53%
Breast Augmentation	1,000	5,500	2,400	18%	82%
Breast Lift	1,000	6,500	2,890	18%	82%
Breast Reduction	1,500	8,000	4,040	19%	81%
Buttock Implants	N/A	N/A	N/A	N/A	N/A
Buttock Lift	1,000	5,000	2,960	57%	43%
Calf Implants	N/A	N/A	N/A	N/A	N/A
Cheek Augmentation	600	4,000	1,760	14%	86%
Chemical Peel				8%	92%
Full-Face	500	3,000	1,640		
Partial-Face	100	1,500	680		
Chin Augmentation				12%	88%
Implant	300	2,500	1,060		
Osteotomy (bone-cut)	600	3,500	1,580		
Collagen Injections	100	500	250	0%	100%
	(per cubic centimeter injected)				
Dermabrasion	300	3,000	1,260	8%	92%
Ear Pinning	750	4,500	1,900	9%	91%
Eyelid Surgery				9%	91%
Uppers Only	600	3,100	1,360		
Lowers Only	600	3,580	1,400		
Uppers and Lowers	1,000	5,000	2,450		
Facelift	1,200	8,000	3,880	20%	80%
Fat Injections	170	1,600	600	0%	100%
Fibrel Injections	150	300	240	0%	100%
	(per cubic centimeter injected)				
Forehead Lift	1,000	4,000	1,980	15%	85%
Gynecomastia	750	4,500	1,970	18%	82%
Hair Replacement				4%	96%
Plug grafts (per plug)	7	60	22		
Strip grafts (per strip)	55	750	365		
Scalp reduction	600	3,000	1,440		
Pedicle flap	1,200	3,500	2,460		
Tissue expansion	1,000	5,000	2,700		
Liposuction	500	5,000	1,480	13%	87%
	(for any single site)				
Nose Reshaping	300	6,000	2,590	14%	86%
Pectoral Implants	N/A	N/A	N/A	N/A	N/A
Retin-A	20	150	45	0%	100%
	(per visit)				
Thigh Lift	1,000	6,000	2,840	46%	54%
Tummy Tuck	1,200	8,500	3,430	75%	25%

KEY: * Lows and highs that represent "outliers" are eliminated.

SEX AND AGE OF 1990 ASPRS COSMETIC PATIENTS

PROCEDURE	SEX		AGES				
	MALE	FEMALE	<18	19-34	35-50	51-64	65+
Arm Lift	5%	95%	1%	10%	48%	32%	8%
Breast Augmentation	0%	100%	1%	65%	32%	3%	—
Breast Lift	0%	100%	1%	34%	56%	8%	1%
Breast Reduction	0%	100%	6%	46%	34%	11%	3%
Buttock Implants	N/A	N/A	N/A	N/A	N/A	N/A	N/A
Buttock Lift	7%	93%	2%	13%	73%	12%	—
Calf Implants	N/A	N/A	N/A	N/A	N/A	N/A	N/A
Cheek Augmentation	24%	76%	2%	51%	36%	10%	1%
Chemical Peel	3%	97%	1%	4%	28%	57%	11%
Chin Augmentation	25%	75%	5%	49%	34%	10%	2%
Collagen Injections	7%	93%	—	14%	54%	28%	4%
Dermabrasion	22%	78%	6%	57%	25%	9%	2%
Ear Pinning	51%	49%	•	•	•	•	•
Eyelid Surgery	16%	84%	—	5%	44%	42%	10%
Facelift	9%	91%	—	1%	27%	59%	13%
Fat Injections	9%	91%	2%	23%	53%	21%	2%
Fibrel Injections	12%	88%	—	17%	66%	16%	1%
Forehead Lift	8%	92%	—	2%	38%	52%	8%
Gynecomastia	100%	0%	26%	54%	15%	4%	—
Hair Replacement	100%	0%	—	33%	57%	10%	—
Liposuction	10%	90%	1%	44%	43%	10%	2%
Nose Reshaping	28%	72%	11%	57%	27%	4%	1%
Pectoral Implants	N/A	N/A	N/A	N/A	N/A	N/A	N/A
Retin-A	7%	93%	1%	17%	45%	29%	8%
Thigh Lift	3%	97%	—	24%	48%	27%	1%
Tummy Tuck	7%	93%	—	19%	64%	15%	2%

Key:
* Ear Pinning: 6 years or < — 20%   19-34 — 21%
  7-12 — 33%   34 or > — 10%
  13-18 — 16%

DEMOGRAPHICS FOR COSMETIC PROCEDURES IN 1990

TOP 3 OVERALL:
1. liposuction
2. breast augmentation
3. collagen injections

TOP 3 BY AGE:

3% 18 or Younger
1. nose reshaping
2. ear pinning
3. breast reduction

32% 19-34
1. breast augmentation
2. liposuction
3. nose reshaping

39% 35-50
1. liposuction
2. collagen injections
3. eyelid surgery

22% 51-64
1. eyelid surgery
2. facelift
3. collagen injections

4% 65+
1. eyelid surgery
2. facelift
3. Retin-A/collagen injections

Courtesy of The American Board of Plastic and Reconstructive Surgery, Inc.

TOP 3
BY SEX: **Females 87%**   **Males 13%**

1. liposuction   1. nose reshaping
2. breast augmentation   2. eyelid surgery
3. collagen injections   3. liposuction

TOP 3
BY REGION: **Pacific 26%**

CA, OR, WA   1. liposuction
2. eyelid surgery
3. collagen injections

South Atlantic 21%

FL, DE, DC, GA, MD, NC, SC, VA, WV   1. liposuction
2. breast augmentation
3. collagen injections

Middle Atlantic 16%

NY, NJ, PA   1. liposuction
2. nose reshaping
3. eyelid surgery

East North Central 9%

IL, IN, MI, OH, WI   1. liposuction
2. nose reshaping
3. breast augmentation

West South Central 8%

TX, AK, LA, OK   1. liposuction
2. breast augmentation
3. eyelid surgery

Mountain 7%

AZ, CO, ID, MT, NV, NM, UT, WY   1. liposuction
2. breast augmentation
3. collagen injections

East South Central 5%

AL, KY, MS, TN   1. breast augmentation
2. collagen injections
3. liposuction

New England 4%

CT, ME, MA, NH, RI, VT   1. collagen injections
2. liposuction
3. nose reshaping

West North Central 4%

IA, KS, MN, MO, NE, ND, SD   1. breast augmentation
2. eyelid surgery
3. liposuction

NUMBER OF PROCEDURES PERFORMED BY AAFPRS MEMBERS

	1986	1988
Rhinoplasty	84,000	99,358
Head/neck tumors	70,000	70,247
Head/neck reconstructive	21,000	41,929
Head/neck trauma	19,800	43,012
Injectable fillers (Zyderm)	44,800	42,529
Blepharoplasty	28,000	38,732
Scar Revision	21,600	30,187
Facial Fractures	23,000	26,711
Facelift	20,000	21,025
Dermabrasion	11,400	15,393
Maxillofacial Surgery	6,400	11,510
Mentoplasty	9,000	14,106
Otoplasty	7,400	10,000
Hair Transplantation	8,100	7,043
Chemabrasion	8,800	11,040
Facial Liposuction	17,900	21,112
Laser (endo & skin)*	29,700	25,939
Birthmarks	15,000	4,242
Forehead Lift	4,500	5,882
Browlift	5,100	6,828
Eyebrows	15,000	3,895
Malar Implant	2,000	3,048
Cleft Lip & Palate	1,600	2,186
Burns	700	751
Orthognathic Surgery	250	1,396

* Laser includes endoscopic and skin laser figures.
  No differentiation between two in 1986 figures.

Source: University of North Carolina
        Practice Management Study

Date: 1989

COSMETIC SURGERY
INFORMATION SERVICE
in affliation with
AMERICAN ACADEMY OF
COSMETIC SURGERY

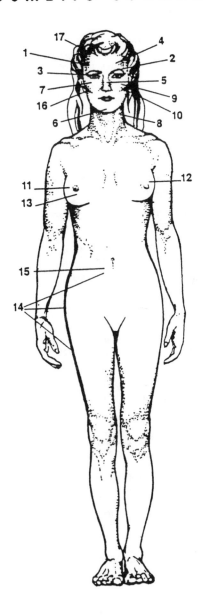

PROCEDURE	RECOVERY TIME	COST
1. FACE LIFT: Skin and facial muscles are tightened and excess skin is removed.	1 1/2- 2 weeks	$3,500-$8,000
2. BROW-LIFT: A section of skin is removed and the eyebrow is lifted.	1 week	1,000-2,000
3. EYELIDS (UPPER/LOWER): Bags, folds and sags in the eyelids are removed. Watery eyes and blurry vision are common short-term side effects.	3 - 10 days	2,000-4,000
4. FOREHEAD-LIFT: Skin is tightened and excess is removed in an "upper" face-lift.	1 1/2- 2 weeks	2,500-4,500
5. NOSE CORRECTION: Length and shape of nose are remodeled to conform to proportions of the face. Difficulty breathing through the nose is a common short-term side effect.	1 week	2,500-6,000
6. CHIN AUGMENTATION: Implants are inserted to enlarge a small or recessed chin.	1 week	1,000-2,000
7. CHEEK (IMPLANTS): Cheekbones are reshaped by insertion of implants.	1 week	1,500-2,500
8. NECK CONTOURING (LIPOSUCTION): Fat cells are removed from neck for contour.	1 week	1,000-2,000
9. CHEMICAL PEEL: The outer layer of skin is chemically treated to remove fine lines or acne scars. Skin may appear pink and blotchy temporarily after treatment.	2 - 3 weeks	2,000-4,500
10. DERMABRASION: Skin is "sanded" to remove fine lines or acne scars. Skin may develop crusts and become pink temporarily after treatment.	2 - 3 weeks	1,000-3,500
11. BREAST AUGMENTATION: An implant is placed in the breast to enlarge size or improve shape.	1 - 2 weeks	2,000-4,000
12. BREAST REDUCTION: Large breasts are reduced in size and made firmer by the removal of excess tissue.	2 - 3 weeks	3,000-6,000
13. BREAST LIFT: The nipple is moved up and breast skin is brought down for support.	1 - 2 weeks	2,000-4,000
14. LIPOSUCTION (FAT REDUCTION): Fat may be suctioned from the thighs, hips, abdomen, knees, face, and under the chin.	2 weeks	1,500-6,000
15. BODY/TUMMY TUCK: Loose skin is tightened and excess skin is removed.	3 - 4 weeks	2,500-6,000

| 16. | **EAR CORRECTION:** The cartilage of protruding ears is reshaped and the ears are pinned back. | 1 week | 1,500-4,500 |
| 17. | **SCALP REDUCTION AND SCALP FLAPS:** Bald skin is moved to improve or correct baldness. | 1 week | 1,000-5,000 |

* Prices may very depending on geographic location and/or severity of the condition.
* Recovery times are average. Individual recovery times may differ.

1) Check into the surgical experience of the surgeon you are considering. Does he or she specialize in the procedure(s) in which you are interested?

2) How many procedures (similar to the one you are interested in) has the doctor performed?

3) How many *cosmetic* procedures is the doctor currently performing per year (per month)?

4) Ask to see before and after photographs, documentation of results or some other proof of artistic ability.

5) The patient should trust and feel that their relationship with the doctor is comfortable.

6) Check into the doctor's background, training and credentials.

7) Recommend that the patient consider more than one doctor, get more than one opinion.

8) Inquire about the risks and benefits of the procedure.

ESTIMATED NUMBER OF COSMETIC SURGERY PROCEDURES PERFORMED BY ASPRS MEMBERS IN 1990

PROCEDURE PERFORMED		TOTAL IN 1990	% CHANGE FROM 1988	% CHANGE FROM 1981
Arm Lift (Brachioplasty)		1,283	N/A	N/A
Breast Augmentation		89,402	+25%	+24%
Breast Lift (Mastopexy)		14,323	+15%	+12%
Breast Reduction		40,258	+13%	+26%
Buttock Implants		100	N/A	N/A
Buttock Lift		783	N/A	N/A
Calf Implants		263	N/A	N/A
Cheek Augmentation (Malar Augmentation)		2,529	− 19%	N/A
Chemical Peel		13,732	+ 46%	+42%
Chin Augmentation (Mentoplasty)		13,333	+ 5%	N/A
Collagen Injections		80,602	+ 17%	N/A
Nose-to-Mouth Lines	51%			
Forehead Frown Lines	37%			
Lip	28%			
Other	10%			
Dermabrasion		16,969	− 16%	no change
Ear Pinning (Otoplasty)		10,159	+ 2%	−12%
Eyelid Surgery (Blepharoplasty)		79,110	+ 1%	+40%
Facelift (Rhytidectomy)		48,743	+0.5%	+25%
Fat Injections		8,220	− 15%	N/A
Nose-to-Mouth Lines	38%			
Forehead Frown Lines	17%			
Lip	21%			
Other	28%			
Fibrel Injections		1,109	− 28%	N/A
Nose-to-Mouth Lines	40%			
Forehead Frown Lines	34%			
Lip	24%			
Other	28%			
Forehead Lift		15,376	+ 4%	N/A
Gynecomastia (Excessive Breast Development in Men)		8,375	N/A	N/A
Hair Replacement (For Male-Pattern Baldness)		3,188	+ 44%	−24%

PROCEDURE PERFORMED		TOTAL IN 1990	% CHANGE FROM 1988	% CHANGE FROM 1981
Liposuction (Suction-Assisted Lipectomy)		109,080*	+ 8%	+95%*
Thighs/Hips	42%			
Abdomen	27%			
Face/Neck	22%			
Legs	9%			
Buttocks	8%			
Nose Reshaping (Rhinoplasty)		68,320	− 7%	+25%
Pectoral Implants (Chest Implants for Men)		139	N/A	N/A
Retin-A		37,338	− 37%	N/A
Thigh Lift		1,221	N/A	N/A
Tummy Tuck (Abdominoplasty)		20,213	− 9%	+32%
ESTIMATED TOTALS		643,910	+ 2%	+69%

Key:

*Liposuction is measured in number of procedures (with each body site considered one procedure), rather than patients, since it is quite common for individuals to have more than one area suctioned at one time during one year. In addition, since liposuction was not introduced to the United States until 1982, statistics were not collected until 1984.

BREAST IMPLANT INFORMATION

from Command Trust Network Newsletter

SOME PROBLEMS AFTER SURGICAL INSERTION OF BREAST IMPLANTS REPORTED TO THE NETWORK

- Shoulder, arm and hand weakness and pain
- Memory loss, word loss
- Burning skin sensations anywhere on the body
- Unusual odor to the urine
- Muscle pain, weakness, burning, spasms, twitches
- Chronic and/or severe headaches
- Drenching sweats, chills
- Nausea, vomiting, irritable bowel syndrome
- Uterine, vaginal and menstrual problems
- Infertility, miscarriage, stillbirth
- Mastectomy due to invasion of breast tissue by silicone
- Surgical removal of chest muscles due to silicone invasion
- Severe emotional toll of multiple surgeries and complications
- Serious lack of resources for psychological and physical help

The newsletter of the Command Trust Network is a clearinghouse of information about breast implants and related issues. To make a tax-deductible contribution or to subscribe to its quarterly newsletter, contact Command Trust Network, P.O. Box 17082, Covington, Kentucky 41017.

Reprinted here with the permission of its authors.

SOME COMPLICATIONS LINKED WITH IMPLANTS IN THE MEDICAL LITERATURE

- Implant rupture
- Multiple surgeries
- Silicone gel bleed from intact implants
- Migration of silicone to nearby tissues and throughout the body
- Connective tissue/autoimmune symptoms and diseases including: Arthritis-like symptoms; Raynaud's phenomenon; Scleroderma; Lupus erythematosus; Sjogren's Syndrome.

These can be painful, crippling, life shortening diseases. Some of the symptoms of these diseases are: joint pain—stiffness—swelling; chronic fatigue; skin thickening and tightening; hardening (fibrosis) and dysfunction or organs and tissues; Vascular (blood vessel) problems; Lung (pulmonary) problems; Sensitivity to cold—sun sensitivity; Dry, burning eyes—dry mouth and nose—vision problems; Anxiety—depression.

MAMMOGRAPHY

Basics: The following guidelines should be followed when obtaining a mammogram:

1) Select a radiologist who does mammograms frequently. It is better to find an office where they do a hundred mammograms a month rather than one that does five or ten a month.

2) In conjunction with the mammogram, a physical examination of the breasts should be performed by the radiologist and not by the technician. The radiologist should be informed of your breast history.

3) Eight views should be taken: 2 compression*, 2 medial displacement cone down views for palpable abnormalities, a contra caudal (top view), right and left contra-lateral (side views), and 2 oblique views (left

and right). Surgical evaluation for a palpable mass is recommended.

*CTN Note: It is possible for compression to cause implant rupture.

XEROMAMMOGRAPHY*

Detecting A Ruptured Implant: Our experts indicate that it may be easier to determine the integrity of an implant, or if there is residual silicone left behind after implant removal, by having a **Xeromammogram**. This technique produces blue ink on white paper.

NEEDED: TWO VIEWS ONLY

1) CONTRA-CAUDAL: Breast horizontal, machine on top. Mild compression of the implant . . . should be comfortable. Do not use machine's pneumatic device. Do not attempt to displace the implant.

2) CONTRA-LATERAL: Side view with machine near the arm. Zero to mild compression of the implant . . . this is comfortable. Gently displace the BREAST to the outside. Try to get small amount of rib cage in the picture. Xeromammography may be performed once a year, until the implants are FOUR YEARS OLD, then every six months after that. RUPTURED IMPLANTS SHOULD BE REMOVED. To locate XEROMAMMOGRAM equipment near you, contact XEROX MEDICAL SYSTEMS (800) 558-6669.

*Xeromammography delivers more radiation to the breast than film screen mammography. Discuss the trade-off with your radiologist.

SONOGRAMS

Some physicians report that sonograms can detect occult (hidden) ruptures. We are not aware of long-term studies about the use of sonograms but it is a process that can be used. We will report more about this when we obtain the information.

EXPLANTATION BREAST IMPLANT REMOVAL: According to CTN reports, breast implant removal after cosmetic breast augmentation leaves some (not all) women looking nearly the same as they did before implant surgery. In some women, breast and/or muscle tissue must be removed to retrieve embedded silicone or polyurethane. Many women with reconstruction also have their implants removed. Some are choosing to rebuild their breasts with their own tissue (called "Flap Reconstruction").

NOTES ON EXPLANTATION (REMOVAL OF IMPLANTS):
In a recent conversation, William Shaw, MD, shared some of his thoughts on the surgical removal of breast implants. Dr. Shaw is the Chairman of the Dept. of Plastic & Reconstructive Surgery at UCLA and has developed the gluteal flap tissue transfer technique of reconstruction. Following are some of the points Dr. Shaw mentioned.

1) There are no absolute answers about explantation because no two cases are alike.
2) It is technically impossible to remove everything. Polyurethane degrades and is irretrievable. Silicone migrates and is irretrievable.
3) A pre-surgical mammogram may be done. Several months after the implants are removed, another mammogram can be done to assure the quality of the explantation surgery.
4) The surgery may require a larger incision to allow for dissecting. There may be more bleeding.
5) Removal of the capsule is a consideration because it is the layer with the greatest residual silicone.
6) General anesthesia is nearly always required if the scar capsule is to be removed.

7) It is sometimes difficult to dissect the implant from the ribs. It takes extra time and there is a greater risk near the ribs and pleura.

8) Where possible the surface of the chest wall should be gone over with a curette.

9) The chest area should be washed with saline solution and an antibiotic wash.

Dr. Shaw saves the implant that has been removed regardless of its condition. It is examined in the pathology department and then can be taken home by the patient. Implants should be sent to a laboratory for independent evaluation.

GENERAL INFORMATION ABOUT EXPLANTATION OF POLYURETHANE IMPLANTS: The latest information from our experts indicates that most of the chemical activity of polyurethane takes place zero to eighteen months after implantation. During this time, it is difficult to remove these "fuzzy" implants.

Option to consider:

1) Have a mammogram to detect the integrity of the implant; an MRI is standard before implant explantation at UCLA. We understand that UCLA has special MRI equipment for this.

2) Ruptured implants should be removed along with surrounding scar capsule.

3) If a polyurethane implant is 18 months to five years old, removal is presumed to prevent further exposure to breakdown products.

4) Tell your doctor to read everything available about polyurethane implants. Search for a surgeon experienced in removing the type of implant you have.

5) Anesthesia options for removing an implant with a silicone outer shell include a LOCAL (with or without sedation) or a GENERAL anesthetic. Discuss these options with the surgeon and the anesthesiologist.

6) Having an implant removed USUALLY involves the same type of pain and recovery time as having an implant put in. Feelings after explantation sometimes include a sense of peace of mind combined with a sense of loss.

7) About two months after implant removal, a mammogram can be performed to see if there is any residual silicone. Some women have chosen to try to have residual silicone removed. This may involve the additional removal of breast tissue, muscle and/or rib tissue.

TESTS

POLYURETHANE FOAM DIAGNOSTIC TESTS MADE AVAILABLE: A method using **Gas Chromatography/Mass Spectrometry** will provide a **POLYTEST ASSAY PROFILE**, which is a procedure for patients with polyurethane foam implants. This testing is being offered by *Aegis Analytical Laboratories, Inc.* of Nashville, Tennessee.

The POLYTEST ASSAY PROFILE is a urine test designed to accurately identify, measure and chart the elimination TDA (the breakdown product of polyurethane known to cause cancer in laboratory animals) if it is present in the body. The test can analytically demonstrate when no TDA is detected. Some scientists have confirmed that TDA can be found in the urine of women up to two years after they have been implanted with polyurethane coated implants. In order to obtain this test:

1) Contact your physician (any with whom you feel comfortable) to discuss your concerns.

2) Request or insist that the physician contact **Aegis Analytical Laboratories, Inc. at (615) 331-5300** to request an appropriate sample collection kit. These specific kits must be used due to the fact that TDA interference might occur from other sample containers.

3) The cost for the **POLYTEST ASSAY PROFILE** kit, analysis of sample and written report is $200. This should be paid to the physician because the test kit will be shipped to the physician C.O.D. Have your doctor tell Aegis Analytical Labs she/he was referred by Command Trust Network.

4) Results will be reported to the physician within seven days of receipt of the sample at the laboratory. Sample shipment to the laboratory by overnight courier is recommended.

5) Testing may be performed on urine (first morning sample is best).

6) THIS TEST CAN BE USED ON BREAST MILK.

INSURANCE BASICS

Many health insurance plans do not want to pay augmentation patients for problems that are considered to be linked to breast implants or for explantation. Mastectomy patients are generally covered for all aspects of reconstructive surgery.

Whether you will recover from your claim the appropriate amount that should be paid according to your coverage largely depends on your own knowledge of your rights and responsibilities.

1) Do your homework before talking to the insurance company. Obtain and read your policies, including declarations and endorsements.

2) Do not speak to any claims representative or insurance company until you have read and understood the parts of the policy that relate to your particular claim.

3) Always take detailed notes of conversations with insurance representatives. Keep records of the date, time, name, position and telephone number of the person with whom you are speaking and summarize the basics of the conversation.

4) Confirm, in writing, the conversations with the representative with whom you have spoken. Be polite and
factually accurate. *Never* exaggerate. Keep copies of all
correspondence.

5) Never give a tape recorded statement or statement
under oath without being certain that you fully understand your legal rights.

Vague, unclear and ambiguous aspects of an insurance policy
must be interpreted in favor of the policyholder. Disability is
defined by the courts and not by the insurance policy.

. . .

Plastic surgeons define a *closed capsulotomy* as breaking the
capsule that surrounds an implant without direct surgical incision. A closed capsulotomy is done by applying direct *external*
pressure to squeeze the implant and its surrounding capsule so
that the capsule cracks and tears. Hopefully the implant remains intact. Breaking the capsule makes the breast feel softer
because the constriction of the capsule is now broken. Complications of closed capsulotomy are:

- Ruptured implant
- Bleeding or hematoma from tissue tearing
- Return of hard capsules
- Severe breast pain
- Damage to physician's hands

Many package inserts warn physicians against performing closed
capsulotomy implant manipulation. Be sure that you read the
package insert that accompanies your implant.

. . .

BREAST IMPLANT
QUESTIONNAIRE

DATE_____

NAME OR INITIALS_____AGE_____

ADDRESS (optional)
_____

1. ARE YOU TOTALLY SATISFIED WITH YOUR BREAST IMPLANTS?
   ___NO   ___YES

2. ORIGINAL BREAST IMPLANT SURGERY:
   ___AUGMENTATION ___RECONSTRUCTION

   DATE_____
   *IMPLANT TYPE (circle) GEL   TX-GEL SAL   TX-SAL   PU   DBL
   **MANUFACTURER
   _____

   IMPLANT PLACED___BEHIND LATISSIMUS DORSI (MUSCLE FROM THE BACK)
                ___IN FRONT OF CHEST MUSCLE
                ___BEHIND CHEST MUSCLE
   DR.'S NAME & LOCATION
   _____

   TYPE OF SURGEON   ___PLASTIC ___COSMETIC   ___GENERAL___OTHER
3. CAPSULAR CONTRACTURES (hardening)?   ___NO ___YES
   CLOSED CAPSULOTOMIES (cracked by hand)?   ___NO ___YES# _____
   OPEN CAPSULOTOMIES (surgery for hardening)?   ___NO ___YES# _____
4. SURGICAL REVISIONS FOR OTHER REASONS?   ___NO ___YES# _____
   REASONS? ___BLEEDING ___DEFORMED   ___IMPLANT SIZE
   ___IMPLANT RUPTURE   ___INFECTION ___OTHER
   _____

   DATES OF SURGICAL REVISIONS
   _____

   *NEW IMPLANTS? (circle any) GEL TX-GEL SAL   TX-SAL   PU   DBL
   **MANUFACTURERS ?
   _____

   TOTAL # OF IMPLANTS
   _____

5. HAVE YOU HAD INFLAMMATION (pain, swelling, redness, heat) OR OTHER
PROBLEMS YOU FEEL ARE DUE TO BREAST IMPLANTS?
_____

_____

6. ARE YOU TAKING NSAIDS (MOTRIN, ADVIL, NUPRIN, ASPIRIN, ETC.)?
_____

7. HAVE YOU BEEN TOLD TO HAVE IMMEDIATE REMOVAL OF A SUSPECTED
RUPTURED GEL FILLED IMPLANT? ___NO   ___YES
8. HYSTERECTOMY?   ___NO   ___YES   DATE
_____

9. WOULD YOU RECOMMEND BREAST IMPLANTS TO YOUR CLOSEST FRIEND
OR DAUGHTER? ___NO   ___YES COMMENTS
_____

10. IF YOU HAVE HAD IMPLANT PROBLEMS, DID YOU REPORT TO THE FDA?
___NO   ___YES

SEND TO:CTN, INC., P.O. BOX 17082, COVINGTON, KY 41017

[Editor's note: If you have breast implants, we would welcome you to participate in this survey by photocopying and completing this questionnaire and sending it to Command Trust Network at the above address. Any information on breast implants is invaluable—KO]

AUGMENTATION MAMMOPLASTY CONSULTATION

Patient Name:_____Age:_____

Chart #:_____

GENERAL:
  Group/Private Exam
    ___Surgery you do not need—Totally/Purely elective surgery—Long consultation
    ___Realistic Expectations - Key to Success

DIAGNOSTIC/CONDITION:
  MAMMARY HYPOPLASIA (small breasts):
    ___Developmental (failure to develop desired fullness and size)
    ___Involutional (loss of size/fullness following pregnancy or significant weight loss)
    ___Unilateral (one breast smaller than the other)

WHY CONSIDER BREAST ENLARGEMENT?
    ___SELF   ___Not for Others

PURPOSE:
    ___Establish more normal proportions
    ___Re-establish size and contour (if size/fullness changed by pregnancy or weight loss)
    ___Maintain normal softness and sensitivity
    ___Maintain function

LIMITATIONS:
    ___Cannot stimulate normal breast tissue to increase in size
    ___Cannot create younger skin or eliminate "stretch marks"
    ___If sagging severe, cannot eliminate with implant alone (options?)

This checklist was written by Dr. Lawrence Seifert as an "informed consent" form, well before informed consent was required by the FDA. Dr. Seifert covered these points in the initial consultations. The patient was asked to check off the items that she did not understand and to call the office for clarification.

___Cannot eliminate asymmetries such as differences in breast shape or position, rib cage irregularities, or nipple/areola size
___Cannot solve personal problems
___GOALS MAY BE ONLY PARTIALLY MET

ALTERNATIVES:
    ___No surgery (adverse consequences)
    ___Exercise
    ___Medications
    ___Surgery
       ___Tissues from somewhere else in the body (autogenous fat or dermal fat grafts)
       ___Synthetic implant
          ___Silicone injection
          ___Silicone implant
          ___Gel (silicone envelope filled with silicone gel)
          ___Inflatable (silicone envelope filled with saline—same as IV solution)
          ___Combination/double lumen (gel implant surrounded by saline or vice versa)
          ___Textured implant (covered with polyurethane or textured silicone)
          ___Implant placement—in front of muscle/behind muscle

INCIDENCE OF CANCER FOLLOWING AUGMENTATION:
    ___Not increased or decreased
    ___Physical examinations not affected since implants placed behind breast tissue NOT in breast tissue
    ___X-rays of the breast (mammograms) require a radiologist experienced in reading mammograms in patients with implants
    ___Mammograms for patients with implants may be more expensive than routine mammograms.
    ___Silicone (as well as many other materials commonly used in human surgery) have been found to cause a very unusual cancer (fibrosarcoma) in laboratory rats—this is not breast cancer—this phenomena appears to be unique to rats—not humans.

SURGICAL TECHNIQUE/ANESTHESIA/FACILITY/RECOVERY:
    ___Local anesthesia & sedation vs general anesthesia
    ___Incisions
    ___Office OR/aesthetic surgical unit/hospital OR
    ___Dressings
    ___Out-patient vs hospitalization
    ___Massage (with smooth wall imp)
    ___Restrictions/return to normal activities

TRADE-OFFS:

Temporary:
___Discomfort (pain/sensitivity)
___Discoloration/Swelling
___Numbness
___Tightness/Relaxation
___Lumps/Irregularities
___Restricted Activity

Permanent:
___Scars
___Tendency toward Firmness
   if Normal Contracture Occurs
___Life Long Need for Follow-up

RISKS/COMPLICATIONS:

___Bleeding/Blood collection**
___Infection
___Sensory changes (numbness)
___Asymmetry
___Implant Failure
___Benign tumors/granulomas
   from gel
___Deflation

___Wrinkling/Irregularity
___Thinning of Overlying Tissue
___Inability to breast feed
___Severe Tightening of Scar Tissue
   Around Implant Producing
   Marked Firmness
___Stretch Marks

___Immune Response (possible allergic reaction—may occur in an extremely small and peculiarly susceptible group of patients—arthritis, fever, malaise, etc., would create suspicion)

LIKELIHOOD OF SUCCESS:

Usually very good—but long term development of abnormal firmness can reduce "natural" feel and affect contour; less than 1% of patients have ever asked to have implants removed.

___EVEN THOUGH THE RISKS AND COMPLICATIONS CITED ABOVE OCCUR INFREQUENTLY, THEY ARE THE ONES THAT ARE PECULIAR TO THE OPERATION OR ARE OF GREATEST CONCERN—OTHER COMPLICATIONS AND RISKS CAN OCCUR BUT ARE EVEN MORE UNCOMMON.

ANY AND ALL OF THE RISKS AND COMPLICATIONS CAN RESULT IN:
___Additional Surgery
___Hospitalization
___Time Off Work
___Expense to You

___INSURANCE USUALLY DOES NOT COVER THE PROCEDURE; TREATMENT OF COMPLICATIONS MAY OR MAY NOT BE COVERED BY INSURANCE.

___LETTER

___NO GUARANTEE—the practice of medicine and surgery is not an exact science; although good results are expected, there cannot be any guarantee, nor warranty, expressed or implied, by anyone as to the results that may be obtained.

** Must be off all aspirin containing products for two (2) weeks before surgery and for two (2) weeks after surgery. (Check all medications with us; some medications such as Motrin and Advil may also affect clotting.)

IF THERE IS ANY ITEM ON THIS CONSULT SHEET THAT YOU DO NOT UNDERSTAND, MARK IT, AND CALL THE OFFICE. AN EXPLANATION OR ADDITIONAL INFORMATION WILL BE PROVIDED. SHARE THE INFORMATION WE PROVIDE WITH YOUR HUSBAND OR OTHER INTERESTED FAMILY MEMBERS OR FRIENDS. I WILL BE HAPPY TO MEET WITH THEM IF YOU WISH.

_____Individual
_____Group_____Primary Consultation_____Same Information as No. _____

Seen In Office Consultation With: (list chart #'s)_____

_____

Date:_____Surgeon:_____

Copy & provided to patient by:_____

A copy of this Consultation was provided to me:_____
                                            (Patient's Signature)

This section of the form was to be completed at the second consultation.

AUGMENTATION MAMMOPLASTY EXAM

Patient Name:_____Age:_____No:_____

CHILDREN: No:_____

Effect on Breasts:_____

_____

PREVIOUS BREAST DISEASE/SURGERY:_____

_____

FAMILY HISTORY OF BREAST CANCER:_____

_____

BLEEDING HISTORY:_____YES_____NO
       IF YES, DETAILS:_____
       MEDICATIONS:_____

LAST MAMMOGRAM:_____

       RESULTS:_____

       WHO HAS REPORT?_____

EXAM
       CURRENT BRA SIZE:_____
       SYMMETRY:
       CHEST WALL CONFIGURATION:
       PTOSIS:
       MASSES/TENDERNESS:
       PREVIOUS SCARS:

<u>DIAGRAMS</u>:

ANY RISKS MORE LIKELY OR SPECIFIC IN THIS PATIENT?

PLAN: CANDIDATE FOR IMPLANT ONLY   YES____NO____
       PTOSIS: _____YES_____NO
       MAMMOGRAM:_____YES_____NO
       INCISION:
       ANESTHESIA: LOCAL_____GENERAL_____
       OVERNIGHT STAY?   YES____NO____
       TO BE DISCUSSED AT TIME OF SURGERY_____
       OTHER:

DATE:_____SURGEON:_____

Reprinted courtesy of Dr. Lawrence Seifert, Los Angeles, California.

LEGISLATIVE EXAMPLES FROM CALIFORNIA

Senate Bill No. 2036

. . .

[Approved by Governor September 30, 1990 . . .]
Legislative Counsel's Digest
SB2036, McCorquodale. Healing arts.

. . .

This bill would provide that a physician and surgeon may include a statement that he or she is certified or eligible for certification by a private or public board or parent association if that board is a specific private board, a board or association with *equivalent* requirements approved by the physician and surgeon's licensing board, or a board or association with an approved postgraduate training program, as specified. This bill would become operative on January 1, 1993, except that certain agencies or organizations could take action contemplated by the bill on or after January 1, 1991.

The people of the State of California do enact as follows:

SECTION 1 . . .
651 (a) It is unlawful for any person licensed under this division or under any initiative act referred to in this division to disseminate or cause to be disseminated any form of public communication containing a false, fraudulent, misleading, or deceptive statement or claim, for the purpose of or likely to induce, directly or indirectly, the rendering of professional services or furnishing of products in connection with the professional practice or business for which he or she is licensed . . .

(b) A false, fraudulent, misleading, or deceptive statement or claim includes a statement or claim which does any of the following:

(1) Contains a misrepresentation of fact.

(2) Is likely to mislead or deceive because of a failure to disclose material facts.

(3) Is intended or is likely to create false or unjustified expectations of favorable results.

(4) Relates to fees, other than a standard consultation fee or a range of fees for specific types of services, without fully and specifically disclosing all variables and other material factors.

(5) Contains other representations or implications that in reasonable probability will cause an ordinarily prudent person to misunderstand or be deceived.

(c) Any price advertisement shall be exact, without the use of such phrases as "as low as," "and up," "lowest prices" or words or phrases of similar import . . . Price advertising shall not be fraudulent, deceitful, or misleading, including statements or advertisements of bait, discount, premiums, gifts, or any statements of a similar nature . . .

(f) Any person so licensed who violates any provision of this section is guilty of a misdemeanor . . .

(g) Any violation of any provision of this section by a person so licensed shall constitute good cause for revocation or suspension of his or her license or other disciplinary action.

(5) . . . A physician and surgeon licensed . . . by the Medical Board of California may include a statement that he or she limits his or her practice to specific fields, but may only include a statement that he or she is certified or eligible for certification by a private or public board or parent association if that board or association is an American Board of Medical Specialties member board, a board or association with equivalent requirements approved by that physician and surgeon's licensing board, or a board or association with an Accreditation Council for Graduate Medical Education approved postgraduate training program that provides complete training in that specialty or subspecialty . . .

Assembly Bill No. 190
January 4, 1991

Legislative Counsel's Digest
. . . Physicians and surgeons: informed consent.

. . .

Existing law makes it a misdemeanor and provides that it is unprofessional conduct to prescribe, dispense, administer, or furnish liquid silicone for the purpose of injecting it into a human breast or mammary.

This bill would require a physician and surgeon to give each patient a copy of the relevant standardized written summary describing the risks and possible side effects of silicone implants, as defined, and collagen injections, as defined, used in *cosmetic*, plastic, reconstructive, or similar surgery, before the physician and surgeon performs the surgery . . .

...

SECTION 1 . . .

2259 . . .

(b) Prior to performance of surgery, the physician and surgeon shall note on the patient's chart that he or she has given the patient the standardized written summary or written information required by this section.

(c) The failure of a physician and surgeon to comply with this section constitutes unprofessional conduct . . .

. . .

(i) . . . "silicone implant" means any implant containing silicone, including implants using a silicone gel or silicone shell. This definition includes implants using a saline solution with a silicone shell.

. . .

SEC. 2 . . .

2259.5 . . .

. . .

(e) . . . the state department shall develop a standardized

written summary to inform the patient of the risks and possible side effects of collagen injections as used in cosmetic, plastic, reconstructive, or similar surgery. In developing this summary, the state department shall do all of the following:

. . .

(3) Identify the type of animal used to produce the collagen and identify the situations where the federal Food and Drug Administration has given its approval for the procedure.

(4) . . .

(i) For purposes of this section, "collagen" includes, but is not limited to, any substance derived from animal protein, or combined with animal protein, that is implanted into the body for purposes of cosmetic, plastic, reconstructive, or similar surgery. However, "collagen" does not include absorbable gelatin medical devices intended for application to bleeding surfaces as a hemostatic or any other medical device used for purposes other than beautifying, promoting attractiveness, or altering the appearance of any part of the human body.